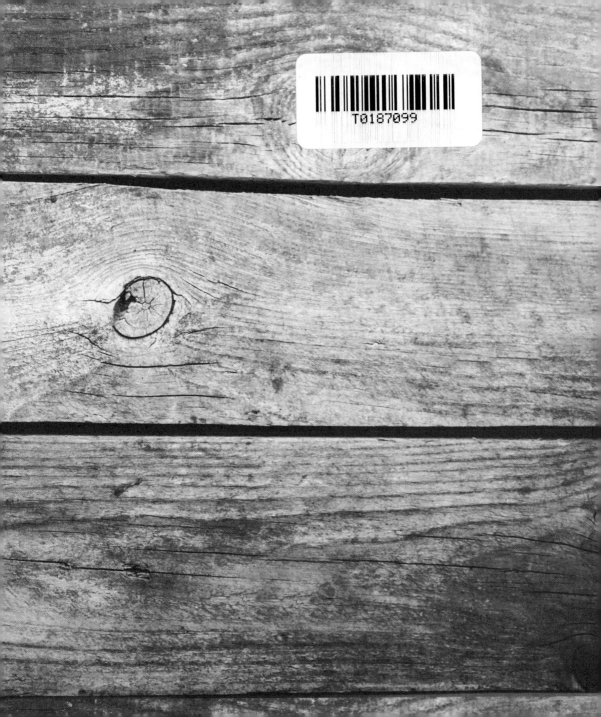

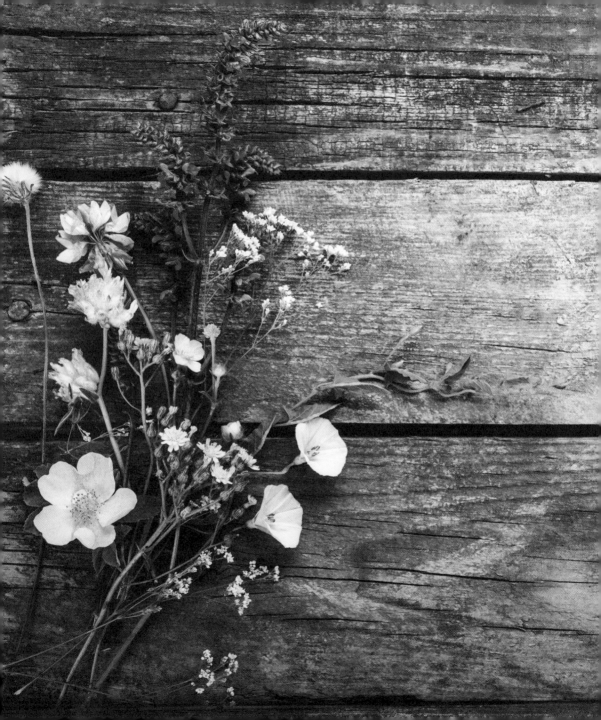

THE
HEDGEROW
APOTHECARY

THE HEDGEROW APOTHECARY

An Hachette UK Company
www.hachette.co.uk

Summersdale Publishers
Part of Octopus Publishing Group Limited
Carmelite House
50 Victoria Embankment
LONDON
EC4Y 0DZ
UK

www.summersdale.com

Printed and bound in China

ISBN: 978-1-78783-029-5

This FSC® label means that materials used for the product have been responsibly sourced

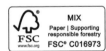

MIX
Paper | Supporting responsible forestry
FSC® C016973

Substantial discounts on bulk quantities of Summersdale books are available to corporations, professional associations and other organizations. For details contact general enquiries: telephone: +44 (0) 1243 771107 or email: enquiries@summersdale.com.

THE
HEDGEROW
APOTHECARY

RECIPES, REMEDIES
AND RITUALS

CHRISTINE IVERSON

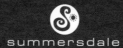

summersdale

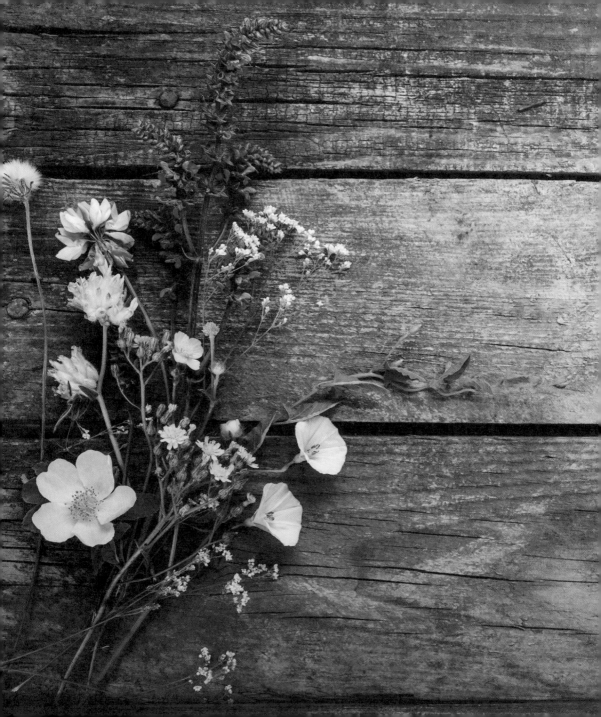

CONTENTS

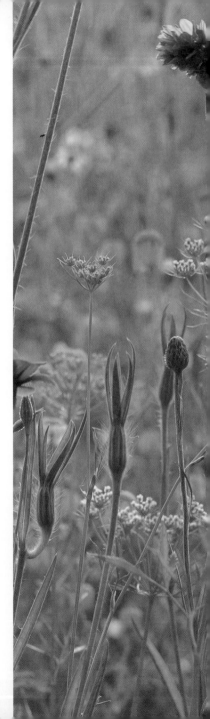

For my wonderful family and friends. Blessed to have your love, support and encouragement.

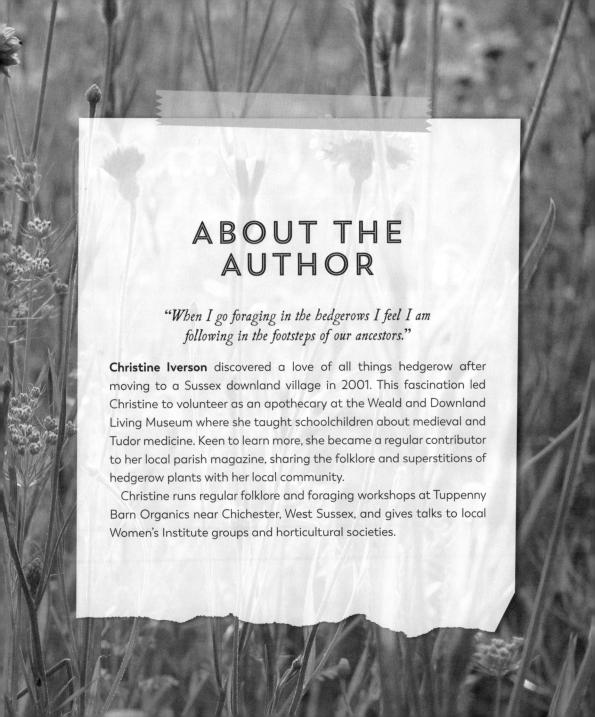

ABOUT THE AUTHOR

"When I go foraging in the hedgerows I feel I am following in the footsteps of our ancestors."

Christine Iverson discovered a love of all things hedgerow after moving to a Sussex downland village in 2001. This fascination led Christine to volunteer as an apothecary at the Weald and Downland Living Museum where she taught schoolchildren about medieval and Tudor medicine. Keen to learn more, she became a regular contributor to her local parish magazine, sharing the folklore and superstitions of hedgerow plants with her local community.

Christine runs regular folklore and foraging workshops at Tuppenny Barn Organics near Chichester, West Sussex, and gives talks to local Women's Institute groups and horticultural societies.

INTRODUCTION

For centuries our ancestors have looked to nature not just for food, but also for healing. Every medieval village would have resident "cunning folk" who would know where to find just the right plant to be turned into a cure for almost anything. As their patients were often poor, they would engage in bartering so that payment might be in eggs or cheese instead of money.

Apothecaries on the other hand were medically trained physicians, who charged a monetary fee for their services. The medieval apothecaries were the predecessors of our modern general practitioners (GPs), often having their own premises in richer towns and cities. An apothecary would give medical advice, and prepare and sell medicines, as well as other products such as wine, herbs and spices. Perhaps the most famous English apothecary was Nicholas Culpeper who upset his colleagues by writing *The English Physician* in the English language instead of the more usual Latin. Culpeper wanted his teachings of medical and pharmaceutical knowledge to be available to everyone.

In a world where medicines and food are available 24 hours a day, 365 days a year from supermarkets, why would you bother to spend your time and energy foraging in the hedgerows? So much of our ancient country knowledge has been lost and I feel passionately that we need to preserve the old ways, and pass them on to the next generation, before they are lost forever. I have noticed a huge resurgence in interest in country ways as people seek a simpler way of life and take more notice of the seasonality and provenance of their food.

I've always loved to make jams and preserves from the fruit given to me by kindly neighbours. Then, in 2001, I moved to a small downland village in Sussex and soon began to notice the fruit all over the hedgerows just begging to be

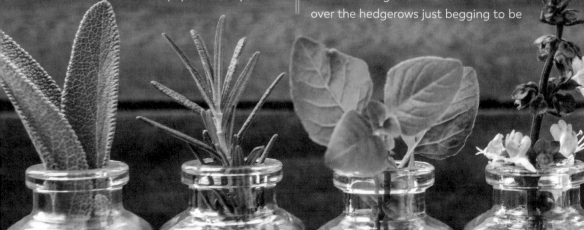

picked. At this point, my foraging knowledge was very limited, but the idea of food for free was just too tempting. I bought a very simple field guide, donned my boots and cautiously began my journey. Beginning with elderberries, I discovered that these plump, black berries could be transformed into a remedy for coughs and sore throats. This proved to be so popular with family, friends and locals in my village that I was soon getting requests to make it every winter. At this time, I was volunteering at The Weald and Downland Living Museum as a Tudor apothecary, running workshops for schoolchildren. This amazing place fired up my imagination and made me want to learn not only about the healing properties of plants, but also the history and fascinating folklore attached to them.

Time spent among nature is never wasted time; studies have shown that our mental health benefits greatly from just being in woodland.

Our ancient hedgerows are being routinely ripped out by housing developers with devastating effects on wildlife corridors and native species; being aware of hedgerows in your locality can help you to protect them. Every walk can be seen as an opportunity to learn, identify a new plant, gather something to eat and, most importantly, reconnect both yourself and your children with nature.

Don't be afraid to forage: begin with something easily identifiable, such as blackberries, to make into vinegar or jam. With the help of this book, you'll soon feel confident to move onto something a little less familiar and the more you look, the more you will find.

It is vital that you take personal responsibility for your safety when foraging. Many plants should not be used during pregnancy, on young children or babies, or on people with certain medical conditions. Consult your GP if you have any doubts.

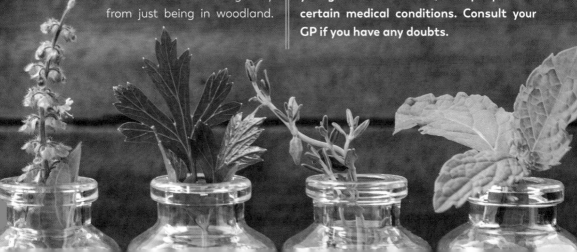

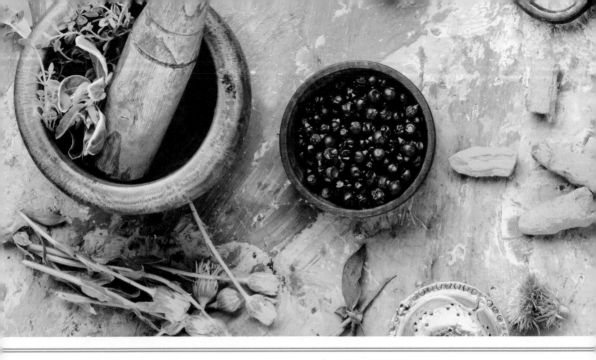

FORAGING TOOLKIT

- A good pocket-sized field guide with clear pictures is essential. If you are not 100 per cent certain that you can correctly identify a plant, DO NOT PICK IT!

- Clothing: you will inevitably encounter nettles and brambles, so long trousers, long sleeves, gardening gloves and sturdy boots are recommended.

- Secateurs or scissors are useful and cause less damage to the plants. I wouldn't advise carrying a knife for safety's sake.

- Baskets are best to transport soft fruit, keeping it in the best condition. And I always like to carry extra bags for those unexpected finds.

- "Hooky stick": My own invention – a long piece of garden cane with a large hook screwed into the end. This will gently pull the higher branches down to you, because the best fruits are always just out of reach! A walking cane will work just as well.

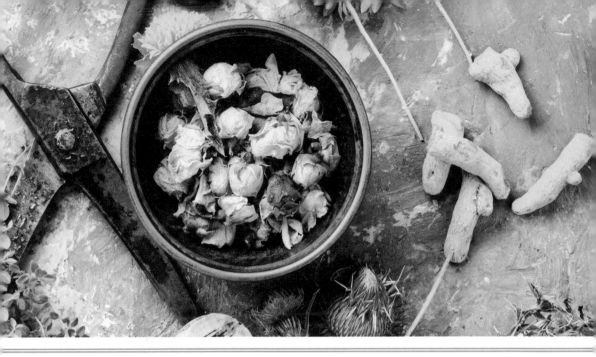

FORAGING ETIQUETTE

🍂 **Location:** If you wish to forage on private land you MUST get permission from the landowner first. I find that the promise of some homemade goodies usually persuades them to welcome your visit. Avoid areas that have been contaminated by road pollution or fields that have been sprayed with pesticides or may have been contaminated by dogs.

🍂 **Respect nature:** Pick no more than you need, leaving plenty for wildlife to enjoy. Try not to disturb habitats and take all rubbish away with you. Stay away from any Sites of Special Scientific Interest (SSSIs) in the UK as these are protected for a reason.

🍂 **Do not pick endangered species:** (Your field guide should help you.) The digging up of roots is frowned upon unless they are abundant and a common species.

🍂 **Be cautious when trying new foods:** Be especially cautious if you have any medical conditions.

🍂 **Share your knowledge:** Teach others how to forage safely and sustainably.

FORAGING CALENDAR

JANUARY, FEBRUARY, MARCH

Chickweed, Common Mallow Leaves, Common Sorrel,
Cowberry, Crow Garlic, Dandelion Root, Garlic Mustard,
Ground Elder, Hairy Bittercress, Nettles, Pignut, Sheep's
Sorrel, Silver Birch Sap, Wild Garlic, Winter Cress, Wood Sorrel

APRIL, MAY, JUNE

Beech Leaves, Borage, Broom, Chickweed, Cleavers,
Common Poppy, Dandelion Leaves and Roots, Dog
Rose Flowers, Elderflower, Garlic Mustard, Ground
Elder, Hawthorn Blossom, Hops, Nettles, Pignuts,
Sheep's Sorrel, Spearmint, Sweet Cicely, Watercress,
Wild Garlic, Wild Thyme, Wood Sorrel, Yarrow

JULY, AUGUST, SEPTEMBER

Acorns, Apples, Beech Nuts, Bilberries, Blackberries,
Burdock, Chamomile, Chickweed, Chicory, Cleavers,
Common Mallow, Dandelion Leaves and Flowers,
Elderberry, Fat Hen, Garlic Mustard, Gooseberries,
Hawthorn Berries, Hazelnuts, Horseradish, Juniper Berries,
Nettle, Plums, Rowan Berries, Sheep's Sorrel, Spearmint,
Sweet Chestnuts, Sweet Cicely, Walnuts, Wild Cherries,
Wild Strawberries, Wild Thyme, Wood Sorrel, Yarrow

OCTOBER, NOVEMBER, DECEMBER

Chestnuts, Chickweed, Crab Apples, Hawthorn
Berries, Horseradish, Nettles, Rosehips, Sheep's Sorrel,
Sloes, Spearmint, Sweet Chestnuts, Walnuts

KITCHEN ESSENTIALS

You don't have to spend a fortune on specialist kitchenware; you can manage well with basic cooking utensils and a little ingenuity. A few large pans are essential, a sieve and colander, and some cotton muslin – although a clean cotton tea towel will work well too. A pestle and mortar if you have one, or a food processor, will make life easier. Jam jars and bottles of differing sizes can be new or recycled, as long as the lids are clean and undamaged, and handwritten labels always look lovely.

Carrier oils: These can be almond oil (don't use if you have a nut allergy), peach kernel oil or even olive oil. These are easily available online and in some health food shops.

HOW TO STERILIZE JARS AND BOTTLES:

1. Wash the jars and lids thoroughly in hot soapy water and rinse.

2. Lay the jars in an oven preheated to 140°C (285°F) for 10–15 minutes until dry.

3. Soak the lids in boiling water in a bowl, then dry thoroughly with kitchen paper before use.

A BRIEF HISTORY OF "CUNNING FOLK"

Other names for cunning folk: Wise Women/Men, White Witch, Charmer, Hedge Witch, Soothsayer

Cunning folk of some description could be found in every medieval village, they could be male or female, young or old, rich or poor. For their services, cunning folk often charged a small fee or an exchange of goods from the poor, and a much higher price from the gentry.

Black magic was thought to come from the devil, whereas the white magic practised by cunning folk was initially regarded by the Church as a "gift from the angels" and, as such, was beneficial. Cunning folk were called upon to heal sickness in both humans and animals, to find and punish thieves, help crops to grow, look into the future, cast horoscopes, tell fortunes and to help people find love. Quite a job description!

Cunning folk were the contemporary experts on preventative measures against black witchcraft and could offer a lot more help in this area than any physician or holy man. They not only offered protective charms and potions, but could also identify and disarm the black witch by using counter-spells.

Bellarmines, or witch bottles, were sometimes used. A bellarmine is a brown ceramic jug usually depicting a face on its side. It was used by witches for capturing spirits, hexing people or to remove curses or hexes. Particularly used by the English west country witches these bottles can last for centuries and are still being discovered in old country houses. In 1644, the Reverend William Brearley lodged in a Suffolk village; his landlady had been ill for quite a while when a cunning man came knocking. Her concerned husband, who was worried that his ill wife had been cursed, was advised by the cunning man to:

"Take a Bottle, and put his Wife's Urine into it, together with Pins and Needles and Nails, and Cork them up, and set the Bottle to the Fire, but be sure the Cork be fast in it, that it not fly out."

Regrettably the cork did fly out and the counter magic was unsuccessful so, when the cunning man returned, he told the husband to "... bury it in the Earth; and that will do the feat." After this, the wife soon recovered to full health.

The educated classes did not always approve of the "gainful trade" of cunning folk and criticized and mocked them, even trying to enforce laws against them.

An illustration of how popular cunning folk were viewed appears in a sermon in 1552 by Bishop Hugh Latimer:

> *"A great many of us when we be in trouble, or sickness, or lose anything, we run hither and thither to witches, or sorcerers, whom we call wise men... seeking aid and comfort at their hands."*

Cunning folk rarely wrote notes about their activities, although luckily some still survive, having been passed down orally.

For example, a cure for thrush was recorded by John Aubrey in his book *Miscellanies* upon various subjects:

> *"Take a living frog, and hold it in a cloth, that it does not go down into the child's mouth; and put the head into the child's mouth 'till it is dead; and then take another frog and do the same."*

And for toothache:

> *"Take a new nail, and make the gum bleed with it, and then drive it into an oak."*

In the sixteenth century across England, many people, mostly women, were accused of witchcraft by members of their local communities and put on trial; the cunning folk very rarely suffered a similar fate.

However, the Witchcraft Act of 1736 refused to accept the existence of magic, and took the opinion that there had never been any real witches, and therefore this new act came down much more heavily on the cunning folk, who were claiming to perform genuine magical spells. It portrayed the cunning folk as practitioners of *"explicitly fraudulent practices designed to fool the credulous"* in order to profit from them. Anyone found guilty *"faced a maximum sentence of one year's imprisonment without bail, and quarterly appearances in the pillory on market days."*

Belief in supernatural power began to decline in the seventeenth century, especially among Puritan authors and more educated members of society. Cunning folk began to be ridiculed and considered to be fraudsters, while black witches were seen as innocent victims.

Sadly, the services of village cunning folk were no longer needed, and records of their work in communities gradually began to vanish from around this time.

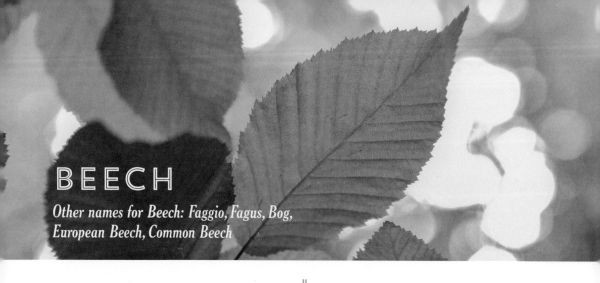

BEECH

Other names for Beech: Faggio, Fagus, Bog, European Beech, Common Beech

HOW TO IDENTIFY: Commonly found growing on chalky soil and beside hedgerows, the elegant beech tree is surely one of the UK's most graceful native trees. It grows to approximately 40 metres (130 feet) tall and is memorable for its large dome-shaped crown and smooth grey bark.

Beech leaves in the spring are soft, smooth and diaphanous, as well as having a delicious lime green hue. By summer, the oval leaves have changed to dark green and the silky hairs seen on the young leaves have disappeared. Autumn's chill turns the leaves a striking copper colour, catching the fading light in the hedgerows and woodlands. Male and female flowers grow on the same tree in spring, followed by catkins producing beech nuts to feed wildlife in the autumn.

HISTORY: The fashionable elegance of the beech tree led to wealthy estate owners planting vast forests of beech in the seventeenth and eighteenth centuries. Unfortunately, they are very shallow rooted and during the great storm of 1987, which hit southern England, many mature trees were either completely uprooted or their roots were weakened so badly that they needed to be felled for safety.

The English word "book" is derived from the Anglo Saxon "*boec*"; beech wood bark is soft and, in Saxon times, was often used to carve writing onto as an early form of book.

Graffiti declaring love can still be seen carved into the bark of beech trees from many years ago, with some messages dating back as far as 250 years. Helen of Troy is even said to have carved the initials of her lover onto the bark of a beech tree.

Some of the many uses for beech wood include: furniture, keels for ships, chairs, clogs and bowls, and it is thought that piles of beech wood were driven into the peaty marshland in Hampshire to make the foundations for Winchester's eleventh-century cathedral.

FOLKLORE: Saint Leonard lived a solitary life in a beech forest on the Sussex/Hampshire border. He had dedicated his life to prayer and cherished the peace and tranquillity of the woodland. Unfortunately, the woods were also inhabited by snakes that disturbed his peace in the daytime and nightingales that kept him awake by singing all night long. Saint Leonard prayed that all the snakes and nightingales would leave the forest so he could enjoy silence once more, and from that time on, neither of these creatures were ever seen again near beech trees.

Known by the Celts as the "tree of wishes", a fallen branch was regarded as an invitation from the faeries to write your wishes on a twig and push it into the soil. Your wish would then be taken into the underworld for consideration by the faery queen.

Prayers said under a beech tree will go straight to heaven and beech bark or leaves carried as a talisman will ensure good luck.

The beech is believed to be nurturing and protective, its canopy gives shade and beech nuts provide nutritious food that can be eaten raw. Lost travellers will come to no harm if they shelter under the branches of the beech tree, though be careful not to swear under the tree or it will drop a branch!

FOLK MEDICINE: Beech leaves have been used to relieve swellings by boiling them to make a soothing poultice. This can be done by heating the leaves in water and wrapping them around the affected area and securing with cloth. The water collected from the hollows of ancient beech trees was thought to cure eczema, psoriasis and many other skin complaints. To speed up the healing of the skin, the patient would sleep on a mattress stuffed with beech leaves.

OTHER COMMON USES:
Beech wood burns well and is traditionally used to smoke herring.

Beech nuts are fed to pigs and can be roasted as a coffee substitute.

Beech trees make a beautiful hedging plant that changes colour with the seasons.

BEECH LEAF NOYAU (LIQUEUR)

I always love the concept of "saving the season" and this simple botanical gin can be made in the spring and then tucked away until Christmas. Pick the bright green young leaves in early spring when they are in plentiful supply.

Makes approximately 1 litre.

INGREDIENTS

1 litre clip-top jar

Enough young beech leaves to loosely fill the jar – gather these away from busy roads

70 cl gin

400 g white granulated sugar

300 ml boiling water

50 ml brandy

METHOD

Pack the jar with leaves then fill it up with gin, making sure that all the leaves are covered as they may turn brown if exposed to the air. Place in a cool, dark cupboard for at least two weeks.

The gin should have taken on a brilliant green colour. Strain the gin through a fine sieve.

Dissolve the sugar in the boiling water and add the brandy. Once cool, mix the sugar syrup into the green gin.

Pour into dark glass bottles; it may turn brown, but this is perfectly drinkable.

Drink neat or over ice with tonic.

Use within one year.

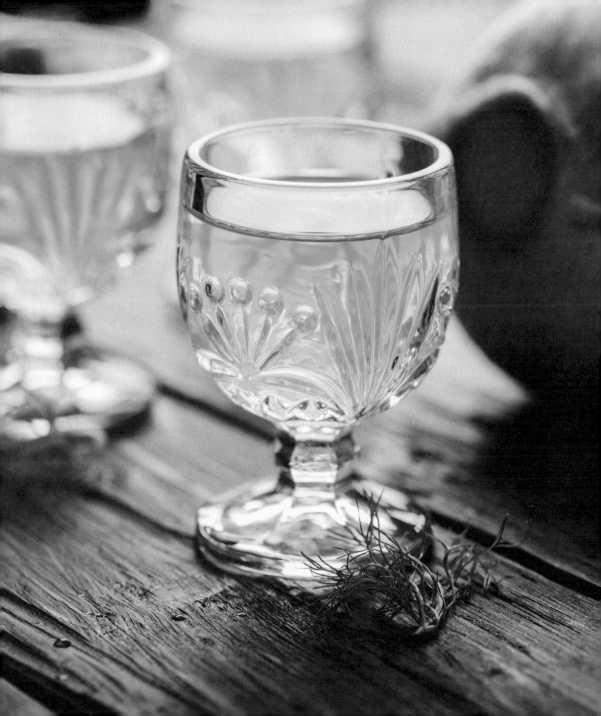

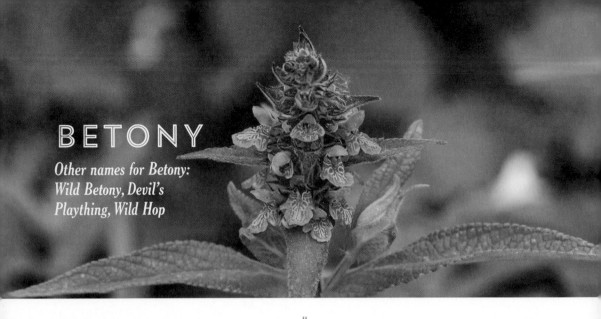

BETONY

Other names for Betony:
Wild Betony, Devil's
Plaything, Wild Hop

HOW TO IDENTIFY: A member of the deadnettle family, betony's bright magenta pink flowers are almost orchid-like and create striking splashes of colour from early summer to well into autumn. Betony can be found growing in light, dry soils on sunny banks and hedgerows or at the edges of ploughed fields. The plant stands up very straight with leaves that are jagged and narrow and mainly found at the base.

HISTORY: Betony was regarded as the most precious remedy used by early European herbalists. Antonius Musa, who was the physician to Emperor Augustus, wrote a book claiming that betony was a cure for no less than 47 diseases.

To demonstrate how valued betony was in the past, the sixteenth-century herbalist, John Gerarde, in his book *The Herball or Generall Historie of All Plantes* (published 1597), recommends that you should:

"Sell your coat and buy betony."

It was widely cultivated in the gardens of apothecaries and monasteries in the Middle Ages and was regarded as a panacea for everyday use.

FOLKLORE: Betony was traditionally planted in country graveyards, not only for its medicinal value, but because it was also believed to ward off evil spirits, ghosts, goblins and any other unwelcome demons.

Betony was added to the water used to bathe children who were alleged to be bewitched or possessed; the bathwater would wash away any bad magic.

Also used as an "amulet herb", betony tied to the arm with red wool or worn around the neck as a charm gave protection from witches, or placed under the pillow at night prevented nightmares and protected the sleeper.

One superstition commonly held during medieval England was that if snakes were placed inside a circle of betony, they would not stop fighting until one of them died.

FOLK MEDICINE: Betony can still be found in English cottage gardens, where it was planted to be used as a home cure for rheumatism and general aches and pains. Betony had the added benefit that growing it around the home would also protect the family from witches and *"terrible goblins that inhabit the night"*.

Wounded wild animals also recognized the benefits of betony and were believed to seek it out to heal themselves.

Traditionally, betony was used to treat mental illness, headaches, insomnia, anxiety, indigestion, nosebleeds, hangovers, memory loss, chest and lung problems and gout, to name but a few. Gerarde also stated: *"It maketh a man to pisse well."*

It was also used to stimulate the uterus and so must be avoided during pregnancy.

OTHER COMMON USES: Betony tea is used by modern herbalists for many complaints such as colds, fevers, poor appetite, sinus trouble and digestive problems.

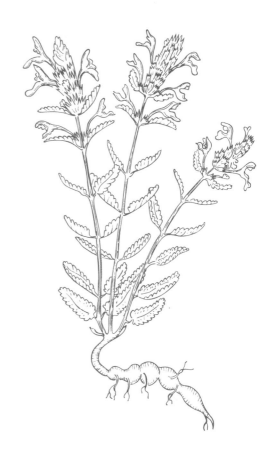

BETONY PICK-ME-UP TINCTURE

If you wake up feeling "just not quite right", betony tincture is a good all-round tonic with numerous healing benefits, such as easing nervous tension and stress, soothing heartburn and digestive problems, headaches and urinary tract infections.

INGREDIENTS

2 large handfuls betony (all parts growing above the ground – stems, leaves and flowers)

Vodka

Jar

METHOD

Simply chop or tear the betony and place it into your jar. If using dried betony, you will only need one third as much as you would the fresh herb.

Pour in just enough vodka to cover.

Place the jar in the dark for six weeks, shaking it occasionally to help infuse the plant into the alcohol.

Strain out the plant material, squeezing it to get the maximum liquid out.

Take one teaspoonful of the tonic up to three times a day.

Keeps for five years.

Always seek your doctor's advice if you are on any medication or have any medical conditions. Not to be used during pregnancy.

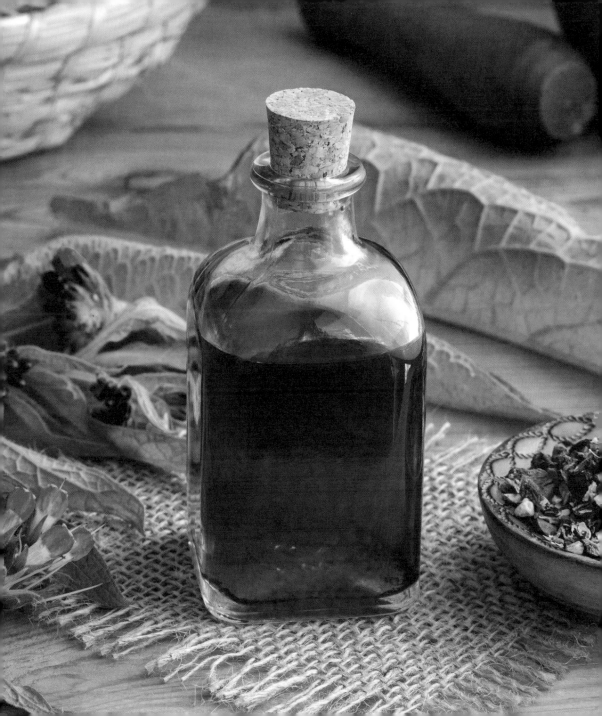

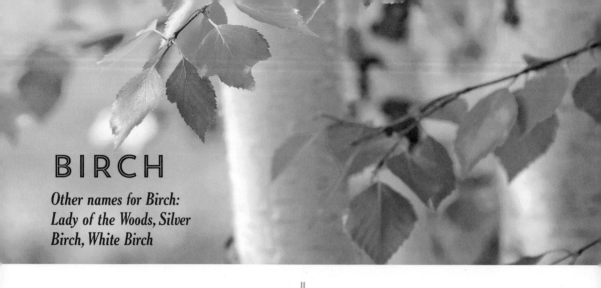

BIRCH

Other names for Birch:
Lady of the Woods, Silver
Birch, White Birch

HOW TO IDENTIFY: With its beautiful silvery-white tissue-paper bark and elegant drooping branches, the birch has a light canopy that allows dappled shade to reach the woodland floor. The leaves are pale green, triangular and small with jagged edges that fade to yellow in the autumn. Attractive yellow catkins appear in spring, changing to dark red with masses of seeds to be distributed on the breeze in autumn.

HISTORY: Known as the oldest tree in Britain, birch appeared when the ice caps retreated and it rapidly colonized the barren land left behind. The thin bark has been used for centuries as writing paper and the trunk hollowed out to make canoes.

Birch twigs can also be tied together to form a makeshift whisk if ever you should need one.

FOLKLORE: In some parts of Britain, the birch would be used as a living maypole to be danced around by villagers on Beltane, the eve of May Day. This is one of the days when witches were believed to be particularly active. Crosses made from birch twigs were hung in doorways to prevent any evil from entering the home. A young birch tree would be felled, wrapped in red and white rags and placed beside stable doors to stop witches from stealing the horses.

Samhain, otherwise known as Halloween, was also a very busy time for witches and the protective properties of the birch were once more called upon. Cradles were fashioned out of birch wood to prevent babies from being bewitched. Dried birch leaves were placed into the cradle too, especially when the child was sick or teething, as they were said to be extremely vulnerable to magic at this time.

FOLK MEDICINE: Dried birch leaves and birch sap are mild diuretics and were used to ease bladder and kidney problems. Skin complaints such as spots and cold sores were treated using a very strong brew of the bark and leaves.

In his book, *Delightes for Ladies*, written in 1609, Sir Hugh Pratt recommends using birch sap for taking away spots and freckles from the face and hands:

> *"The sap doth perform most excellently and maketh the skin very clear."*

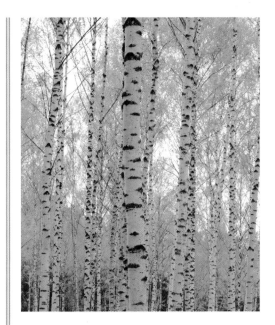

OTHER COMMON USES: Birch sap was prized for its sticky, sweet, delicate flavour, which must have been very welcome to our ancestors after a long winter of very bland food. Tapping is done in early spring using a mature birch tree. With a sterile drill bit, drill a hole about 1 metre (3 feet) from the ground, angling the drill slightly upward – the hole should be about 5 mm (¼ inch) in diameter. Insert some sterile tubing into the hole and catch the sap in a clean container as it flows out. Don't be greedy, only take what you need, then gently remove the tubing and press on the wound until it stops flowing. The sap doesn't stay fresh for long, so use it quickly to make wine, syrup or a soothing skin wash.

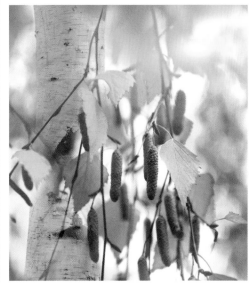

BIRCH LEAF OIL

Collect the leaves in spring and early summer, and turn them into a lovely soothing massage oil to ease aching muscles, reduce cellulite and calm skin affected by psoriasis or eczema.

INGREDIENTS

Fresh young
birch leaves

1 litre jar

Carrier oil (sweet
almond, peach
kernel, for example)

Cotton muslin cloth

METHOD

Put the birch leaves into the jar and cover them with your chosen carrier oil. Cover with a piece of cotton cloth, secured with a band or string.

Place on a sunny windowsill, shaking occasionally to ensure that the leaves stay submerged in the oil.

After a month, the healing properties will have leached into the oil. Strain the mixture through a fine sieve into a jug.

Any water will settle to the bottom of the jug. Carefully pour the oil into sterilized glass bottles, while trying to avoid adding any of the water.

Store away from direct sunlight.

Use within one year.

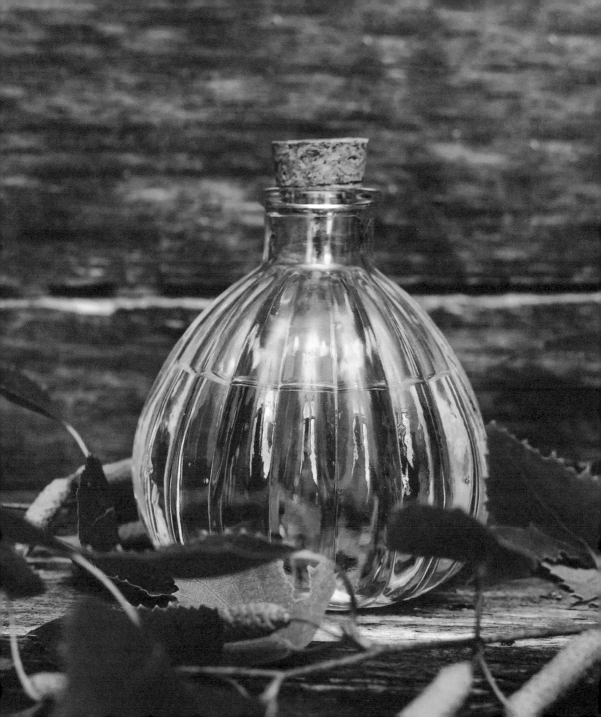

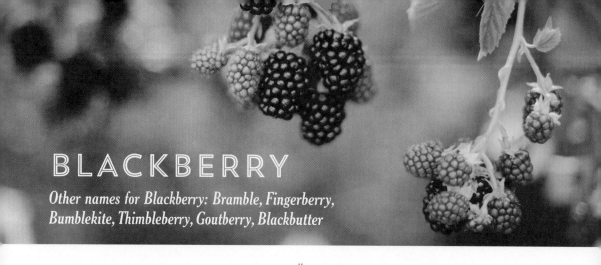

BLACKBERRY

Other names for Blackberry: Bramble, Fingerberry, Bumblekite, Thimbleberry, Goutberry, Blackbutter

HOW TO IDENTIFY: A prickly shrub with white or pink five-petalled flowers; it grows abundantly in the hedgerows and woods from late summer to early autumn. The plump berries turn from green to red to black. The berry at the tip of the thorny stalk is the sweetest of them all, as this is the first to ripen.

HISTORY: The Anglo Saxon name for the plant was *"brymbel"*, which means "prickly". In more recent history, it was nicknamed "lawyers" as an old English proverb says: *"once they get their hands into you, it's not easy to get shot of them."*

Bramble is commonly used as a hedging plant to discourage trespassers.

FOLKLORE: When the devil was thrown out of heaven on Michaelmas Day for his proud and arrogant ways by Archangel Michael, he fell to Earth and landed on a bramble bush. He cursed the plant for pricking him and spat on the fruit, turning them sour and making them inedible. Thus, traditionally blackberries are never picked after Michaelmas Day because they will be sour.

Blackberry bushes were often planted around windows and doors to keep demons out because it was believed that demons were fascinated by counting things; they would feel compelled to count the berries until sunrise, keeping them outside and the family safe inside.

FOLK MEDICINE: Sometimes the long brambles bend over and root at the tip, forming a natural archway. This arch was used in folk medicine for many years to treat boils, rheumatism, whooping cough and hernias. The patient would be passed through the arch to symbolize a new beginning. A baby with whooping cough would be passed through the arch backward from east to west and then three times forward before breakfast for nine consecutive days while saying:

"In bramble, out cough, here I leave the whooping cough."

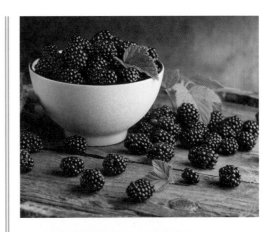

According to *Healing Charms in Use in England and Wales 1700 to 1950* by Owen Davies, in order to soothe a burn, you should collect nine bramble leaves (historically, using ingredients to the power of three was always considered to be a more effective cure), float them in a bowl of either holy or spring water, and then pass the leaves over the burned area three times while saying the following:

"There came three angels out of the East, One brought fire and one brought frost, Out fire and in frost! In the name of the Father, Son and Holy Ghost"

OTHER COMMON USES: The fruit can be used to make a slate-blue natural dye, while the roots give an orange colour that can be used to dye wool and cotton. The fruit can also be used to make delicious jams, jellies, crumbles and wine.

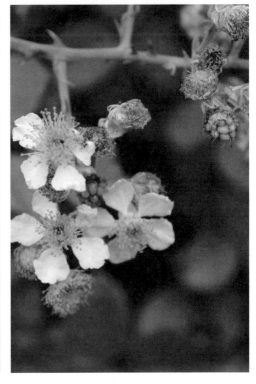

WILD BLACKBERRY VINEGAR

Blackberries are an excellent source of the powerful antioxidant vitamins A, C and K. At the first sign of a prickly sore throat, take a spoonful as a gargle to ease symptoms. It also makes a delicious salad dressing when mixed with an oil of your choice, or use two teaspoons when making meringues to give a chewy texture. Collect your blackberries on a dry day from a hedgerow away from busy roads.

Makes approximately 500 ml.

INGREDIENTS

300 g blackberries

300 g caster sugar

300 ml white wine vinegar

METHOD

Rinse your blackberries in cold water and pat dry with a clean tea towel, allowing any little bugs to escape. Put the berries into a large jar or bowl and cover with white wine vinegar until they are just floating. Cover and place somewhere cool for five to seven days, stirring every day to release the lovely purple colour.

At the end of that time, strain the vinegar from the berries through a fine sieve into a jug. Allow the liquid to gently drip through overnight.

Measure the vinegar and pour it into a large saucepan. For every 100 ml of vinegar, add 50 g of caster sugar and slowly bring to the boil, stirring constantly to dissolve the sugar. Bring to a rolling boil for 5 minutes.

Allow the liquid to cool for 10 minutes, pour into sterilized bottles, cap tightly and label.

Use within one year.

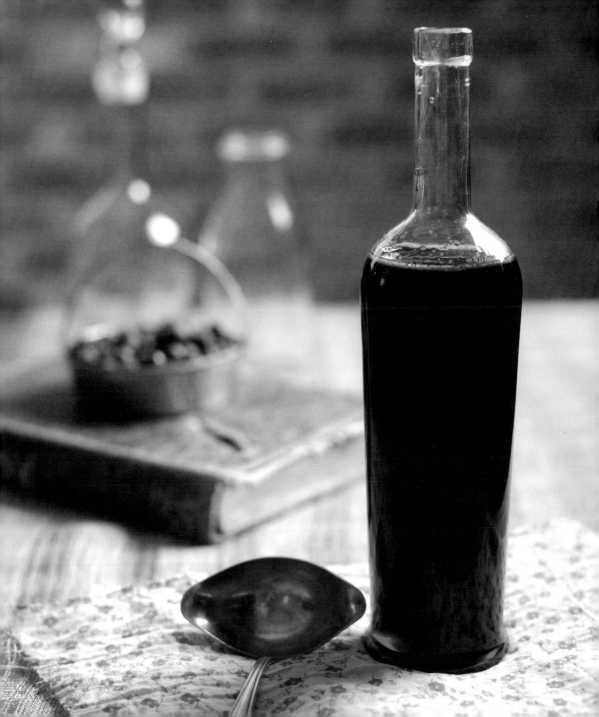

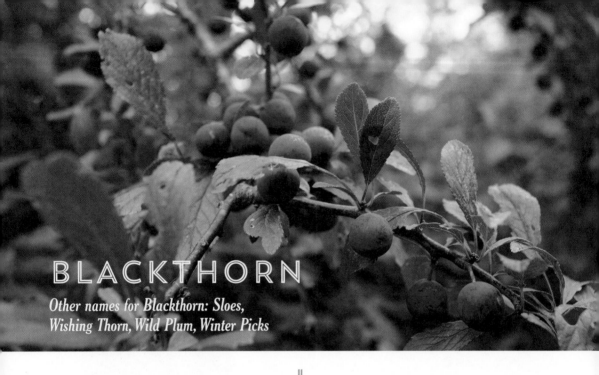

BLACKTHORN

Other names for Blackthorn: Sloes,
Wishing Thorn, Wild Plum, Winter Picks

HOW TO IDENTIFY: The snowy white flowers of the blackthorn are one of the first blooms of spring in the hedgerow. The blackthorn can grow to over 3 metres (10 feet) tall. It has thorny branches, small oval-shaped leaves and purple marble-sized fruits, commonly known as sloes.

HISTORY: Blackthorn in bloom was considered to be an emblem of both life and death together, as the blossom appears when the tree has no leaves. It blooms so early in the year that country folk have always called a spell of cold weather at the end of spring "the winter of the blackthorn".

Traditionally, the blackthorn in full bloom was an indication to farmers that it was the right time of year to sow barley.

FOLKLORE: It was believed that Christ's crown of thorns was made from blackthorn and so to bring blackthorn blossom into the home meant certain death. It is also said that if the blackthorn and the hawthorn have many berries then the following winter will be very cold.

In south Devon folklore witches were said to carry blackthorn walking sticks with which they caused much local mischief. Divining rods, used to search for underground water, were made from two pieces of blackthorn wood that had been cut from the bush between sunset and sunrise on a new moon. The nasty long sharp thorns were used by witches to pierce poppets made into the image of an enemy that they wished to harm.

In medieval times, the devil was said to prick his followers' fingers with the thorn of a blackthorn tree.

FOLK MEDICINE: A popular cure for boils was to crawl around a blackthorn tree backward three times while the morning dew was still on the grass.

Slugs or snails were rubbed onto warts, and then the poor creature would have been impaled on a thorn of a blackthorn tree. As the slug shrivelled and died, so would the warts.

Nicholas Culpeper tells us that:

> *"The fruit is chiefly used for sore mouths and gums and to fasten loose teeth."*

The flowers and fruit were also used to make a tonic for diarrhoea, whitening teeth and as a cure for nosebleeds, constipation and eye pain. Unripe sloes were also used as a very effective purge.

G. Clarke Nuttall reminds country people of the value of foraging for sloes in his 1920 poem:

> *"At the end of October,*
> *go gather up the sloes.*
> *Have thou in readiness plenty of those.*
> *And keep them in bedstraw,*
> *or still on the bough.*
> *To stay both the flux of*
> *thyself and thy cow."*

OTHER COMMON USES: The best use for sloes by far is sloe gin!

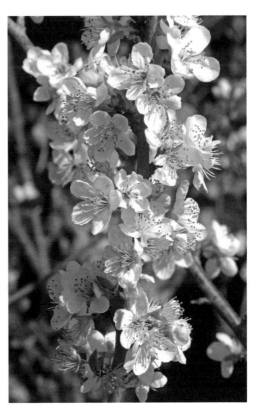

SLOE GIN

INGREDIENTS

500 g sloes (I like
to freeze mine for a
couple of days to burst
them in order to get
the maximum amount
of juice and colour)

250 g caster sugar

70 cl gin (this
doesn't have to be
an expensive one)

METHOD

Put the sloes and the sugar into a sterilized 1 litre jar and pour
over the gin.

Shake well to dissolve the sugar.

Store the jar in a dark cupboard for at least two months,
remembering to shake the jar occasionally.

Sieve out the fruit and decant the liquor into clean bottles. (keeping
the sloes to make sloe port – see below).

You will be rewarded with a stunning scarlet liquor just in time
for Christmas!

SLOE PORT

This uses up the sloes left over once you have made sloe gin.

INGREDIENTS

The sloes that you
have used to make
your sloe gin

70 cl red wine (I
like to use claret)

100 g caster sugar

200 ml brandy

METHOD

Put the sloes, wine and caster sugar into a 1 litre jar and shake
to dissolve the sugar. And into the dark cupboard, once again!

Leave for three weeks, giving it a little shake now and then when
you remember.

After the three weeks, add the brandy, shake well and leave for
at least three months before straining.

As with sloe gin, there's a fair bit of waiting around before you
can sample your sloe port but, believe me, it's well worth it!

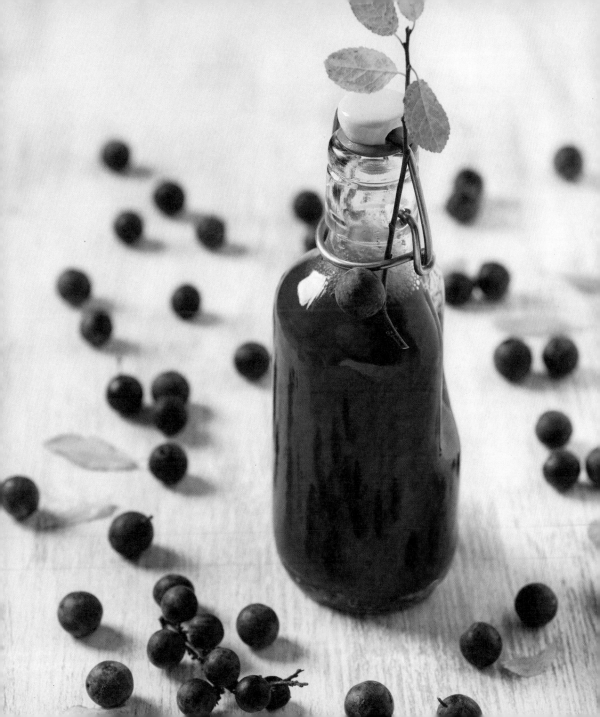

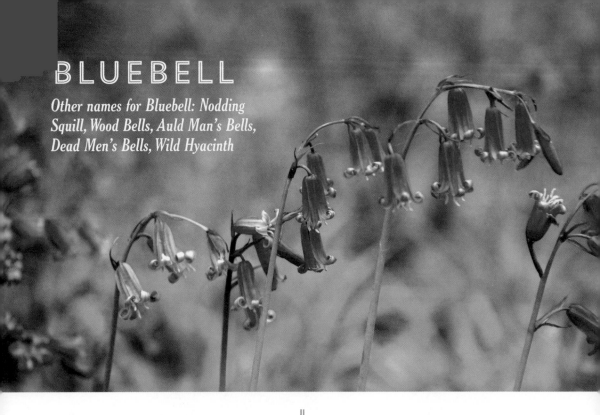

BLUEBELL

Other names for Bluebell: Nodding Squill, Wood Bells, Auld Man's Bells, Dead Men's Bells, Wild Hyacinth

HOW TO IDENTIFY: The English bluebell flower is a deep violet blue in colour, has creamy white pollen and is bell shaped with rolled back tips. The flowers are almost always on one side of the stem, causing them to droop over like a shepherd's crook. Sadly, in recent years, there has been an increase in the non-native Spanish bluebell, which has been imported to grow in domestic gardens. The Spanish bluebell can easily cross-breed with our native bluebells, diluting the purity and jeopardizing our historic bluebell woods. Spanish bluebells can be tricky to recognize, but they tend to be paler in colour with larger flowers, the stems are straight rather than nodding and they have little or no scent.

HISTORY: Bluebell woods have declined over the last century due to competition with other plants and the loss of suitable habitats, however, nearly 50 per cent of the world's bluebells can still be found in the UK. Because bluebells spread very slowly, they're considered to be an indicator of ancient woodland sites. During the Victorian times, bluebell trains once ran through the Chiltern Hills taking city-dwelling tourists on a journey to view the wonderful carpets of bluebells.

Apart from being a plant that delights us with its beauty, the sticky bluebell sap has been used by people in a variety of ways: Bronze Age hunters used bluebell glue to attach feathers to their arrows, bluebell bulbs were crushed to provide starch for the ruffs of Elizabethan and Victorian collars and sleeves, bluebell sap was used to bind pages to the spines of books as it is so toxic that it stopped insects from attacking the bindings.

FOLKLORE: A bluebell wood is an especially dangerous place for families as the faeries will use the bluebells to trap you and kidnap little children.

At dawn, the bells can be heard ringing to summon all the faeries back from their slumbers in the woods, but if a human hears the bells they will be visited by a malevolent faery and die soon after. Not surprisingly, it was considered unlucky to trample on a bed of bluebells because you would surely anger the faeries resting there.

Thankfully not all the bluebell's folklore is quite so scary. Some believed that by wearing a wreath made of the flowers, the wearer would be required to tell only the truth. Others thought that if you could turn one of the flowers inside out without tearing it you would eventually win the heart of the one you love.

Cunningham's Encyclopedia of Magical Herbs recommends that if you are in need of some good fortune, place a bluebell in your shoe while saying:

> *"Bluebell, bluebell, bring me some luck before tomorrow night."*

To dream of bluebells means that unfortunately you are married to a nagging spouse, but that happily your relationship is also passionate.

Place bluebells into your sleep pillow (see also "Mugwort", page 118) or hang them by the bed to help prevent nightmares.

Bluebells were often planted on graves as they represented rebirth and would give comfort to grieving relatives.

FOLK MEDICINE: Bluebells were said by herbalists to help prevent nightmares, and were used as a remedy against leprosy, spider bites and tuberculosis.

Be careful, the bluebell is highly poisonous.

Bluebells are protected under UK law with fines of up to £5,000 per bulb if you are caught digging them up.

BLUEBELL-SCENTED REED DIFFUSER

Nothing is more uplifting than walking through woodland in spring and catching the scent of wild bluebells, so bring the bluebells in with this easy-to-make reed diffuser.

INGREDIENTS

Clean glass bottle with a narrow neck

60 ml carrier oil

30 drops bluebell fragrance oil (available online)

Handful of reed sticks

METHOD

Pour carrier oil into the bottle and then drip in the bluebell fragrance oil and give it a swirl.

Add your reed sticks.

After a couple of hours, turn the reeds upside down in the jar to help the oil travel up the stick.

You can use any essential oils that you wish for this diffuser and it is much more economical than the shop-bought version.

As bluebells are a protected species, when making our reed diffuser we use the bluebell fragrance oil which is a synthetic blend so as not to harm any bluebells. It is also worth noting that bluebells are protected by the Wildlife and Countryside Act (1981). The Act prohibits anyone from digging up bulbs in the countryside and landowners from removing bluebells from their land for sale. The species was also listed on Schedule 8 of the Act in 1998 which makes trade in wild bluebell bulbs or seeds an offence. It is also illegal to pick and sell their flowers.

It is best to enjoy bluebells in their natural environment and to be sure to refrain from picking any of their flowers or accidentally treading on any part of the leaves or stems. This will help to give these beautiful springtime flowers the best chance of sustaining their populations in our ancient native woodlands.

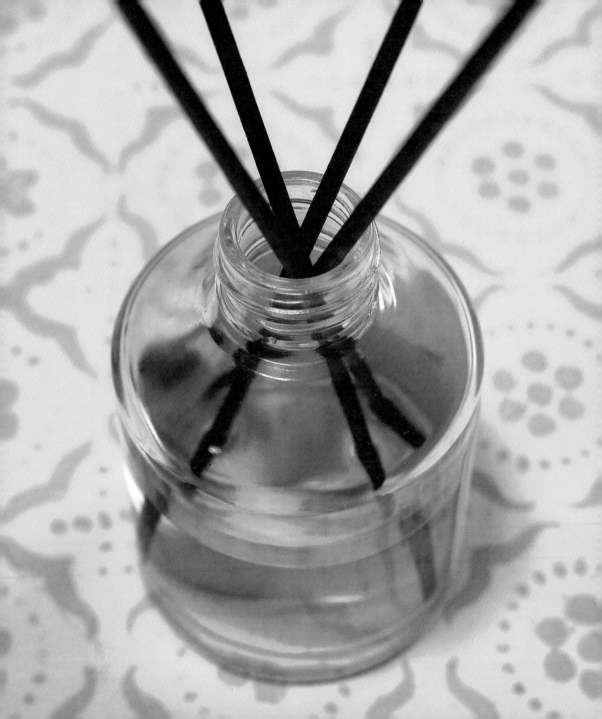

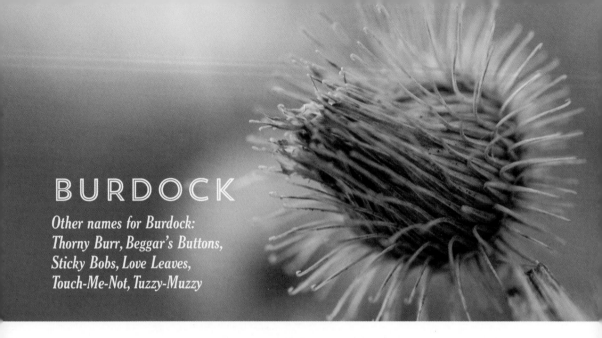

BURDOCK

Other names for Burdock:
Thorny Burr, Beggar's Buttons,
Sticky Bobs, Love Leaves,
Touch-Me-Not, Tuzzy-Muzzy

HOW TO IDENTIFY: A large plant with a long taproot, which is brown or black on the outside. Outsized, wavy, heart-shaped leaves are green on the top and whitish underneath and can measure up to 50 cm (20 inches). Purple, thistle-like flowers bloom between June and October, which then turn into hooked seed-bearing burrs that irritatingly tangle themselves into animal fur and clothing.

HISTORY: The burdock root was much prized by our ancestors as it was one of the first fresh foods available to them after the long, hard winter. To use as a tonic to cleanse the liver and remove toxins, it is best harvested in early spring before the plant flowers as this is when it contains the maximum quantity of antioxidants.

While out walking with his dog, the Swiss engineer, George de Mestral noticed pesky burrs had attached themselves to his dog and his clothing. He put the burrs under a microscope and noticed that they had a hook and loop system, allowing the seeds to hitchhike onto the fur of passing animals. These annoying sticky burrs gave him the inspiration to invent Velcro.

FOLKLORE: Since 1687, on the second Friday in August, a "Burry Man" has been known to parade along the streets of South Queensferry in Scotland, dressed from head to toe in the sticky burrs of the burdock plant. He has to walk 7 miles (11.3 km), which takes him about 9 hours, but he is well rewarded for his efforts with a tot of whisky drunk through a straw in each local pub that he enters. It is believed that he will bring good luck to the town if they give him whisky and money and that bad luck will result if the custom is ever discontinued.

In Midsummer, the plant was picked and placed on buildings to ward off lightning and also braided into hair as protection against evil. During the waning moon, burdock root was dug up, cut into small pieces, dried and made into a necklace as protection against evil.

FOLK MEDICINE: Culpeper used burdock for many illnesses including "bitings of serpents". Mixed with salt as a poultice, it could:

> *"ease the pain of being bitten by a mad dog"* and *"The juice of the leaves, taken with honey, provokes urine and remedies the pain in the bladder".*

The large heart-shaped leaves of the burdock were steamed and used as a hot poultice to wrap around wounds and bruises and to ease the pain of rheumatism, arthritis and gout.

Henry VIII's syphilis treatments appear to have been both numerous and widely varied. Unfortunately, it was never cured, although one of the more palatable treatments involved using burdock leaves mixed with wine.

In medieval times, burdock root oil was a popular cure for baldness.

OTHER COMMON USES: It is still used by modern-day herbalists, who have discovered it to have antibacterial and antifungal properties.

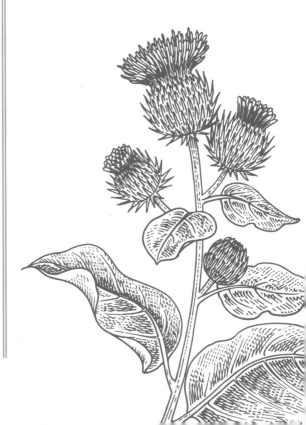

DANDELION AND BURDOCK CORDIAL

Dandelion is high in vitamins A, B, C and D as well as iron and zinc, while burdock is high in fibre with antibacterial, anti-inflammatory and antioxidant properties – perfect for a health-giving treat.

Makes approximately 800 ml.

INGREDIENTS

600 ml cold water

1 tsp ground
burdock root

1 tsp ground
dandelion root

2 cm piece
ginger, sliced

1 whole star
anise, crushed

½ tsp citric acid

300 g granulated
sugar

200 ml soda
water, to serve

METHOD

Place all of the ingredients, except for the sugar and soda water, into a large saucepan and boil for 20 minutes.

Filter the mixture into a serving jug, through a sieve lined with a tea towel or muslin cloth. While the mixture is still hot, stir in the sugar until dissolved. Leave the mixture to cool.

To serve, add 200 ml of soda water to every 50 ml of syrup in a jug and stir well. Pour over ice in glass tumblers.

For an alcoholic version, replace the soda with tonic water and gin.

The syrup will keep in the fridge for six months.

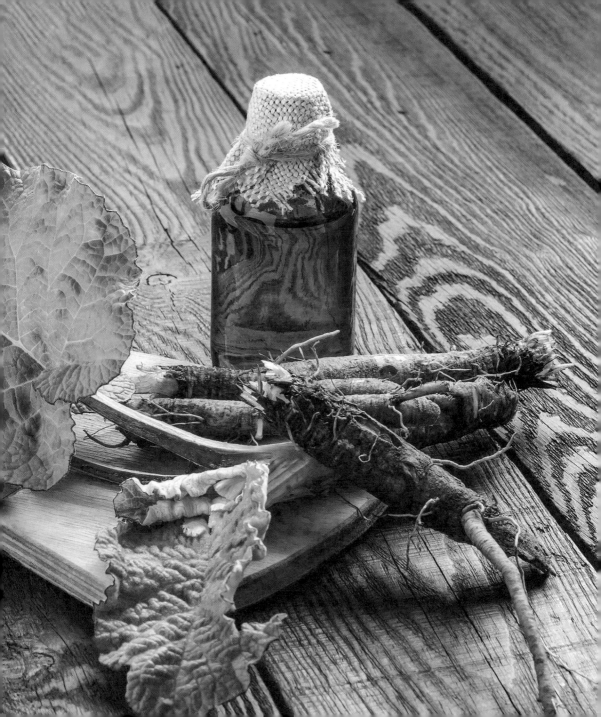

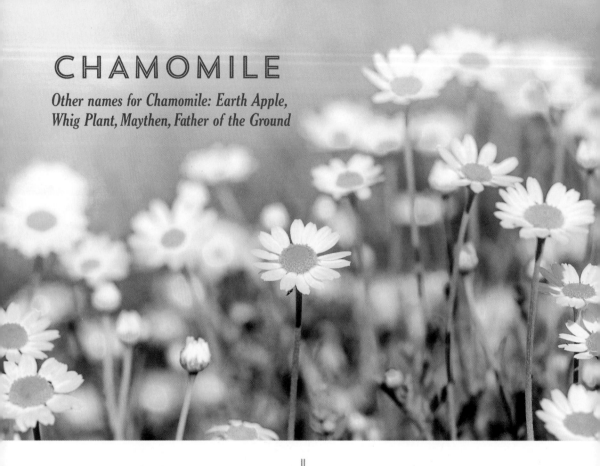

CHAMOMILE

Other names for Chamomile: Earth Apple, Whig Plant, Maythen, Father of the Ground

HOW TO IDENTIFY: A small, creeping plant with daisy-like flowers and feathery leaves. One of the best ways to identify chamomile is to crush it between your fingers and smell – it should have a pleasant, fresh, apple scent.

HISTORY: With its fragrant scent, chamomile was often used as a "strewing herb" on the floors of medieval dwellings.

When it was crushed underfoot, a delicious scent would be released to hide the more unpleasant smells that were common at the time. It was also grown to make sweet-scented seats and lawns in medieval gardens, as well as being prized for its healing properties.

Maud Grieve tells us how to help cultivate chamomile in her book, *A Modern Herbal*, first published in 1931:

"Like a chamomile bed,
The more it is trodden,
The more it will spread."

Found in abundance in the English cottage garden, even Peter Rabbit drank chamomile tea to settle his stomach after eating too many lettuces.

FOLKLORE: Used as a hand wash by gamblers, chamomile was said to ensure good luck and attract money. Bathing in chamomile will help to attract true love. Plant chamomile near windows and doors, as this will prevent negativity from entering your home. Carry some in your pocket if you ever think you might be in danger of magical or physical attack.

FOLK MEDICINE: Culpeper prized this soothing herb:

"It moderately comforts all parts that
have need of warmth, digests and
dissolves whatsoever has need thereof,
by a wonderful speedy property."

Grandmother Huggett, who was a nineteenth-century Sussex cunning woman, had a cure for toothache using chamomile and poppies:

"Ah, and if you happen to be plagued
with toothache — I used to be fair terrified
of it when I were a girl — you need a
nice warm poultice of poppy seeds and
chamomile flowers boiled up together.
Takes the pain away wonderful that do!"

OTHER COMMON USES: Bunches of chamomile plants can be hung in open windows to keep flies away. Chamomile infusion makes a lovely rinse to bring out the colour in blonde hair. Of course, chamomile tea has long been used to help relax and get a good night's sleep.

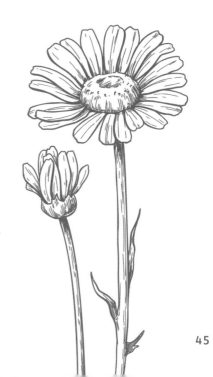

GENTLE CHAMOMILE HAND SCRUB

With its gentle, exfoliating action and the strong anti-inflammatory properties of chamomile, this scrub will soothe hard-working hands, leaving them soft and smooth.

Makes approximately one 225 g jar.

INGREDIENTS

4 tbsp vegetable glycerine – you can find this in the baking aisle of the supermarket

30 g cornflour

4 tsp ground rice

4 tsp finely ground oats

2 tsp freshly made chamomile tea

METHOD

Warm the vegetable glycerine in a heatproof bowl over a saucepan of boiling water.

Add the cornflour slowly and stir until a paste is formed.

Take the bowl off the heat, still stirring, and slowly add the chamomile tea.

Mix in the oats and ground rice.

Store in a labelled sterilized jar and use within two months.

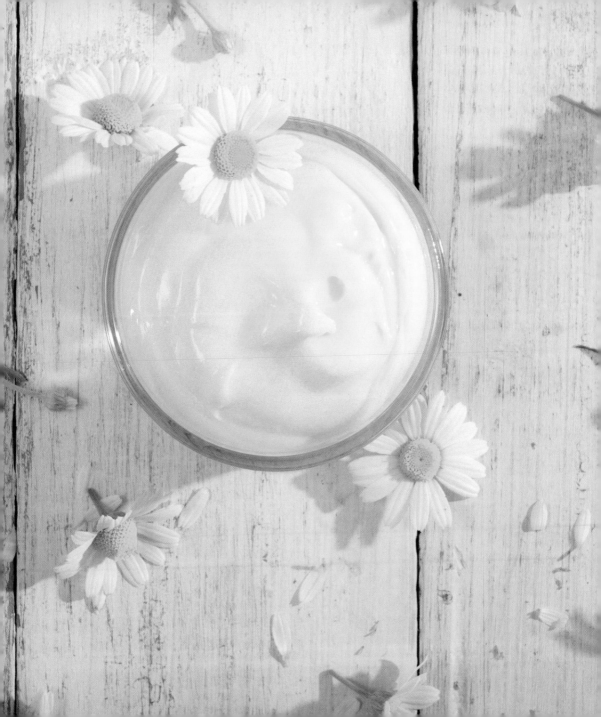

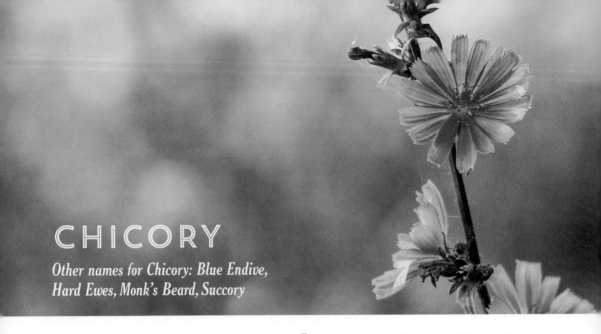

CHICORY

Other names for Chicory: Blue Endive, Hard Ewes, Monk's Beard, Succory

HOW TO IDENTIFY: The straggly stems of the chicory plant are bedecked with multiple blue, daisy-like flowers from July to October. The large-lobed leaves look similar to dandelion leaves with deep lobes growing smaller toward the tip. Branching stems are covered in fine hairs and have a milky sap inside. Chicory grows in chalky soil and roadside ditches, as well as the disturbed ground at the edge of ploughed fields.

HISTORY: Chicory was used by the Greeks and Romans as a salad plant, a vegetable and as a medicine, and it is one of the first plants to have been mentioned in poetry by the Roman poet Horace:

"Olives, chicory and blue mallow are enough for me to live on."

FOLKLORE: An attractive maiden, whose beauty had captivated the sun, refused its advances and to escape she turned herself into a wild chicory plant. This is why the blue flowers turn their heads to follow the sun as it passes across the sky every day.

On St James Day, 25 July, chicory can be used to open locked doors and cupboards; this must be done in absolute silence. Hold a golden knife and chicory leaves up to the lock and it will open for you. According to tradition, carrying a sprig of chicory will also open doors into unseen worlds and even help you to forget past loves.

Generally believed to bring good fortune, especially to travellers going on an expedition, it was understood to have been carried by prospectors following the gold rush in North America in the eighteenth century.

FOLK MEDICINE: In the eighteenth century, a lady from Peebles, Scotland, had a very interesting use for chicory; plastic surgeons please take note:

> *"For a woman that hath great breasts; Oftentimes anoint her paps with the juice of the succory (chicory), it will make them round and hard: If they be hanging or bagging, it will draw them together, whereby they shall seem like the paps of a maid."*

The flowers of chicory respond to the position of the sun; even on a sunny day every bloom is closed by midday, having opened at 6 or 7 a.m. It was therefore thought that distilling the flowers into eye drops would make an effective remedy for failing eyesight. Chicory was used for loss of appetite, rapid heartbeat, constipation, upset stomach and jaundice.

Nicholas Culpeper gives us an insight into early seventeenth century medicine and how he used chicory in his London apothecary practice:

> *"The distilled water of the herb and the flowers is especially good for hot stomachs, and in agues, either pestilential or of long continuance, for swooning and passions of the heart, for the heat and headache in children and for the blood and liver."*

OTHER COMMON USES: Chicory leaves can be used to make a blue dye. In the kitchen, chicory leaves can be added to salads and also used as a cooking spice.

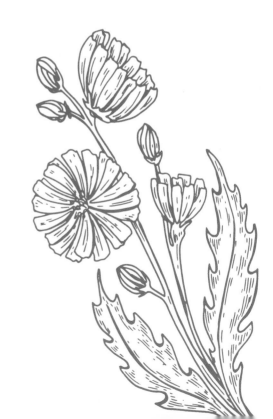

CHICORY MOCHA

It is believed that chicory coffee originated during a massive coffee shortage in France in the 1800s when people, desperate for their coffee fix, began using chicory root as a substitute. As well as being naturally caffeine free, chicory also contains manganese and vitamin B6, which is essential for brain health.

Makes one large mug.

INGREDIENTS

2 tbsp roasted chicory root powder (available online)

250 ml water

250 ml milk or milk substitute

1 tbsp cocoa powder

1 tsp maple syrup

Whipped cream (optional)

METHOD

Combine the chicory powder and water in a small saucepan, bring to the boil, simmer for 10 minutes, then strain into a jug.

In another saucepan, combine the milk, cocoa powder and maple syrup. Whisk over a low heat until fully combined. Don't let it boil.

Add the strained chicory root coffee to the cocoa mix and warm through.

Top with whipped cream for an indulgent treat.

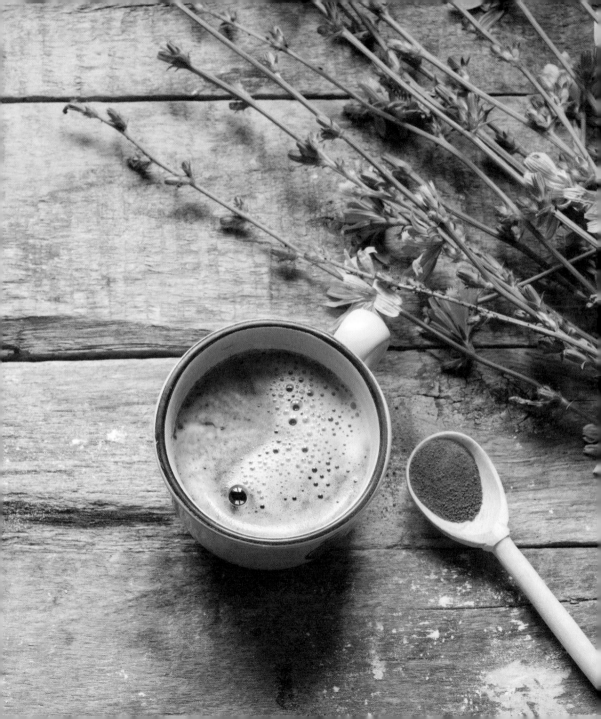

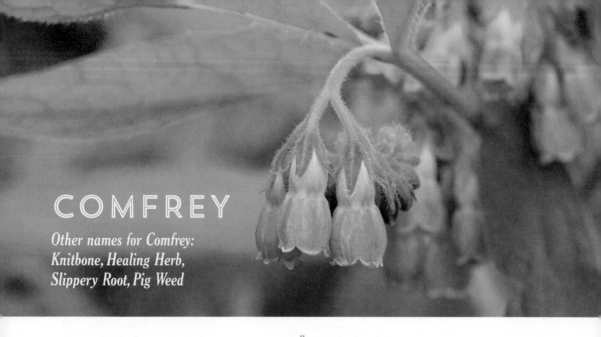

COMFREY

Other names for Comfrey:
Knitbone, Healing Herb,
Slippery Root, Pig Weed

HOW TO IDENTIFY: Comfrey grows in damp, shady woodlands and hedgerows. It is quite easy to spot with its broad, lance-shaped hairy leaves, similar to foxglove leaves. Be careful as this can fool novice foragers with deadly consequences as foxglove leaves are toxic! Clusters of pink, purple or white trumpet-shaped flowers begin to appear in May, dangling on the end of thick, hairy stems.

HISTORY: The name comfrey derives from the Latin "*conferre*", meaning "come together", and has been grown for its bone-healing properties since about 400 BC. The Romans and Greeks recorded how they used comfrey to heal broken bones, stop heavy bleeding and treat lung problems. Medieval herbalists dug up the roots in spring and grated them to make "nature's putty", which was packed around a broken limb. The putty then hardened, immobilizing the broken bone in a way similar to plaster of Paris today. The allantoin contained in comfrey helped prevent infection, promoted new cell growth and helped to heal the break.

A medical trial in America in 2005 compared the effectiveness of comfrey cream with diclofenac gel in treating sprained ankles. The group using comfrey reported significantly less pain and swelling.

FOLKLORE: Travellers would carry comfrey in their possessions to prevent them from being stolen or lost. Wearing comfrey in shoes not only kept the traveller safe but ensured that their partner stayed faithful while they were gone.

FOLK MEDICINE: Young ladies wishing to restore their "maidenhood" were often advised to take a bath with comfrey in the hope that its healing powers would make them virgins once again.

Culpeper was clearly a fan of comfrey, claiming that if the roots:

> *"Be boiled with dissevered pieces of flesh in a pot, it will join them together again."*

Furthermore, he recommends comfrey for:

> *"Spitting, pissing blood, inward wounds and bruises... muscles cut, wounds, ruptures, broken bones, knotted breasts, haemorrhoids, inflammation, gout..."*

Many early herbalists used comfrey leaf tea to treat bronchitis and other chest complaints, while Gerarde advises that it should be:

> *"given to drinke against the paine of the back, gotten by violent motion as wrestling or overuse of women."*

Benedictine and Cistercian monks grew vast amounts of comfrey in the monastery gardens as they would be expected to treat the wounds of soldiers returning from many conflicts.

OTHER COMMON USES: Comfrey ointment can be purchased in most health food shops.

Still used as medicine and by smallholders for their cattle and chickens.

Using comfrey internally is NOT recommended.

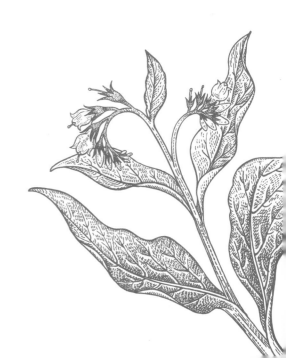

COMFREY LEAF PLANT FEED

Why use chemical fertilizers when it is so simple to make an environmentally friendly and nutritious organic feed at home for free? Comfrey feed is rich in potassium, making it perfect for tomatoes, flowers and fruits, and you can make enough to keep you going all year round.

INGREDIENTS

Comfrey leaves

Large bucket or tub

Old plastic
milk bottles

METHOD

Wear gloves to harvest the hairy leaves from the bottom of established plants.

Remove any tough stems and flowers before roughly chopping the leaves and packing them tightly into your container.

Place a brick or large stone on top of the leaves and cover with water (rainwater is best if you have it).

Leave for two to four weeks. As the leaves break down, they will release a brown smelly liquid. You want it to resemble weak tea.

Collect the brown liquid in plastic bottles and store in a cool, dark place. It must be diluted before use – as a guide, use one part comfrey feed to ten parts water.

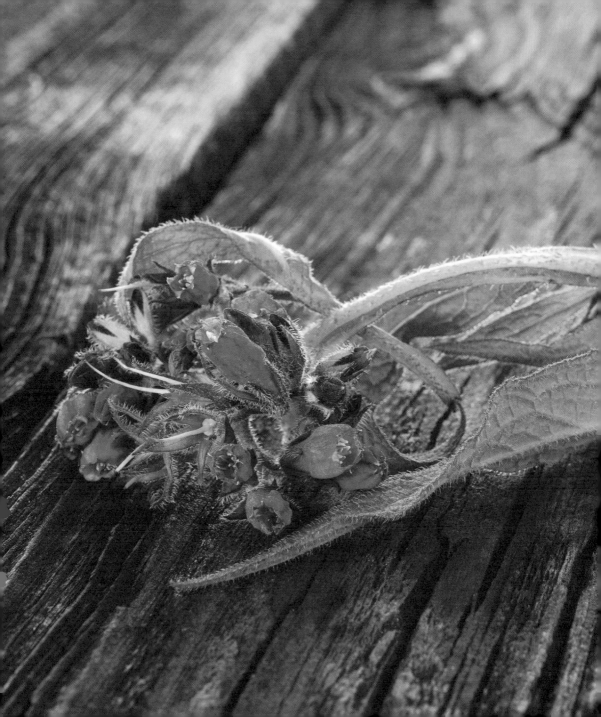

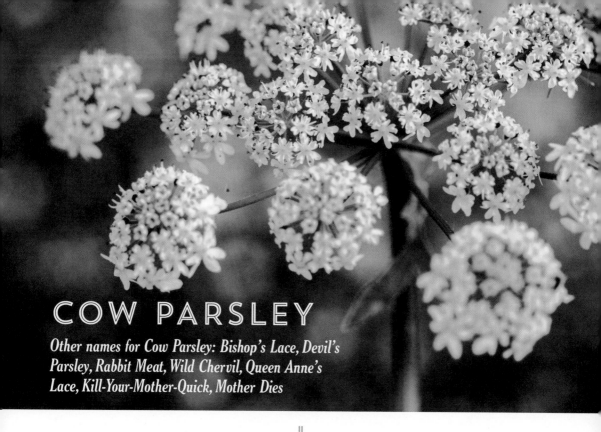

COW PARSLEY

Other names for Cow Parsley: Bishop's Lace, Devil's Parsley, Rabbit Meat, Wild Chervil, Queen Anne's Lace, Kill-Your-Mother-Quick, Mother Dies

HOW TO IDENTIFY: Cow parsley is prolific along country lanes in the springtime. Its umbels of white, frothy flowers are held up by hollow, furrowed stems that grow to about 1.2 metres (4 feet) tall. The leaves are much divided and resemble ferns.

It is easily mistaken for the poisonous hemlock!

HISTORY: It is eaten by cattle, sheep and pigs, hence its name. A glorious range of dye colours can be obtained from the flowering tips of cow parsley including orange, green, yellow and bronze. In the Outer Hebrides (or Western Isles of Scotland), this was put to good use by the locals to dye wool for the famous Harris Tweed fabric.

As Queen Anne travelled the countryside in May to ease her asthma, it was said that the roadside verges had been decorated just for her with lots of pretty cow parsley. The lace pillows that were carried by her ladies in waiting also resembled the delicate flowers of the cow parsley so the plant became commonly known as "Queen Anne's Lace".

FOLKLORE: As with many white-flowered plants, cow parsley is considered to bring bad luck, misfortune or even death if ever taken into the house.

The country names of "Mother Dies" and "Kill-Your-Mother-Quick" illustrate how children were fiercely discouraged from picking cow parsley. The plant is very similar to the highly poisonous hemlock plant, which is deadly.

Bring cow parsley home and snakes will surely follow!

FOLK MEDICINE: A tea is said to treat water retention, help wounds to heal and calm skin eruptions and to treat laminitis in horses.

OTHER COMMON USES: Fresh or dried cow parsley adds interest to flower arrangements and it is often seen planted at the back of cottage garden borders.

The common name for cow parsley is "wild chervil" and it is sometimes used as a substitute for "garden chervil" in cooking.

Applied directly to the skin, cow parsley is an excellent insect repellent.

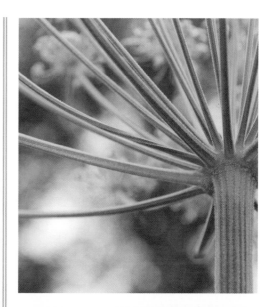

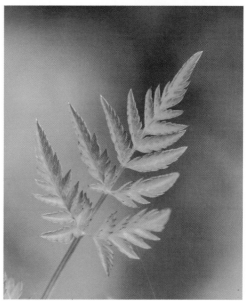

SPRING WREATH

What better way to welcome spring into your home than this delicate pretty door wreath.

YOU WILL NEED

A pre-made wicker wreath (use your old Christmas one if you have one)

Lots of freshly gathered cow parsley

Florist wire or string

Spring foliage and blossom such as blackthorn, primroses, and ivy, for example.

METHOD

Choose where the top is going to be and begin to weave your foliage in through the wicker base. Make sure you overlap everything for a generous covering of foliage. Tie in place as needed, while keeping the string or wire hidden.

Carefully work your way around the wreath until it is completely covered.

Tie a piece of cord around the top so that you can hang it from your door.

I love the way that you can change this wreath to match the seasons: a combination of autumn leaves with pine cones looks fantastic, as do roses and peonies in the summer.

Door wreaths aren't just for Christmas!

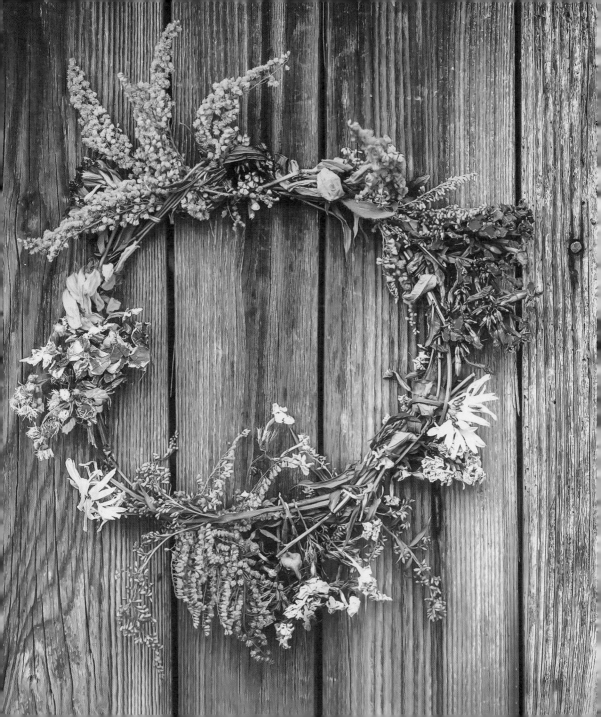

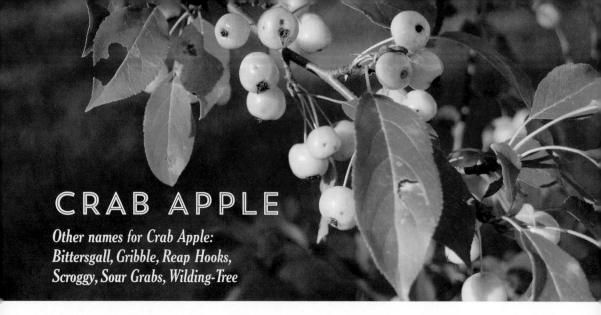

CRAB APPLE

Other names for Crab Apple:
Bittersgall, Gribble, Reap Hooks,
Scroggy, Sour Grabs, Wilding-Tree

HOW TO IDENTIFY: This wild, native species is a diminutive thorny tree that can be found in woodland edges and hedgerows. The deciduous leaves are arranged alternately on the branches and can vary in shape but are roughly oval or round with a pointed end and finely serrated edges. As the tree grows older the scaly, greyish bark becomes cracked, twisted and gnarly. The five-petalled pink flowers bloom in the hedgerow in spring, usually between April and May. Crab apples are sharper and smaller than cultivated apples and may be green, yellow or red in colour. The stalk is long in relation to the size of the fruit when compared to a standard size apple. Their bitter, dry-tasting nature makes them unpalatable to eat but their intense apple flavour works well in many recipes, including drinks and jams.

HISTORY: The crab apple is our only indigenous apple species. It actually belongs to the Rose family along with Hawthorn, Blackthorn and Wild Pear, which all have thorns on their branches. In the eighteenth century, hybrids were brought over from Europe. These were grafted onto wild trees and eventually gave us greater fruit-yielding trees with no thorns: the apple tree as we now know it was born.

FOLKLORE: A woman who married an inferior husband was believed to have gone to the orchard and selected the crab. Conversely, in Scotland, girls would put crab apples under their pillows on St Andrew's Eve (29 November), and then take the apple to church with them. The first man they saw in the church porch was destined to be their husband. Crab apples have long been associated with love and marriage. It was said that you should throw the pips into the fire while saying the name of your love, if the pips explode then your love is true. Apple wood was burned by the Celts during fertility rites and festivals, and Shakespeare makes reference to crab apples in *A Midsummer Night's Dream*:

"And sometimes lurk I in a gossip's bowl,
In very likeness of a roasted crab,
And when she drinks, against her lips I bob,
And on her withered dewlap pour the ale."

FOLK MEDICINE: Crab apple juice is known as "verjuice" and was used for treating sprains, cramps and also as a laxative. Poultices of rotten apples were used on boils, sore eyes and to cure earache. Warts were rubbed with a crab apple which was then buried, taking the wart with it. Smallpox victims had an apple placed in their bedroom, the apple would become spotty and the patient would recover.

Unicorns are believed to live under crab apple trees – keep your eyes peeled!

OTHER COMMON USES: Today, crab apples are used as a pollinator for other fruits.

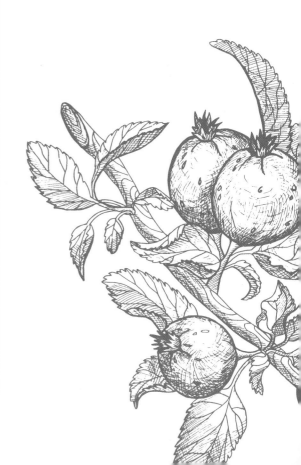

HOT CRAB APPLE AND CHILLI JELLY

From a health perspective, crab apples are a natural antioxidant and high in vitamin C. Their seeds and core are naturally high in pectin making them useful to set jellies and jams. This jelly is a tasty accompaniment to sausages or cold meats, and delicious on toast and crumpets too.

Makes three 500 g jars.

INGREDIENTS

600 g crab apples washed and chopped (I like to use red-skinned ones as they give the jelly an amazing colour)

35 g chopped chillies – go as hot as you dare!

1 litre water

Juice of 1 lemon

500 g caster sugar, approximately

METHOD

Put the chopped apples, chillies, lemon juice and water into a heavy-bottomed pan.

Bring to the boil and simmer for about 30 minutes, until the apples become pulpy.

Strain through a jelly bag or muslin square overnight. Don't be tempted to squeeze the pulp – this would make your jelly cloudy.

Measure the juice into a pan. For every 500 ml of juice add 300 g of caster sugar. Bring slowly to the boil, stirring to dissolve the sugar. Keep a rolling boil going for 10–15 minutes until setting point has been reached.

Cool slightly, skim away any scum that forms on top of your jelly, pour into sterilized jars and seal tightly with screw-top lids.

Keeps for about one year. Refrigerate once open and use within one month.

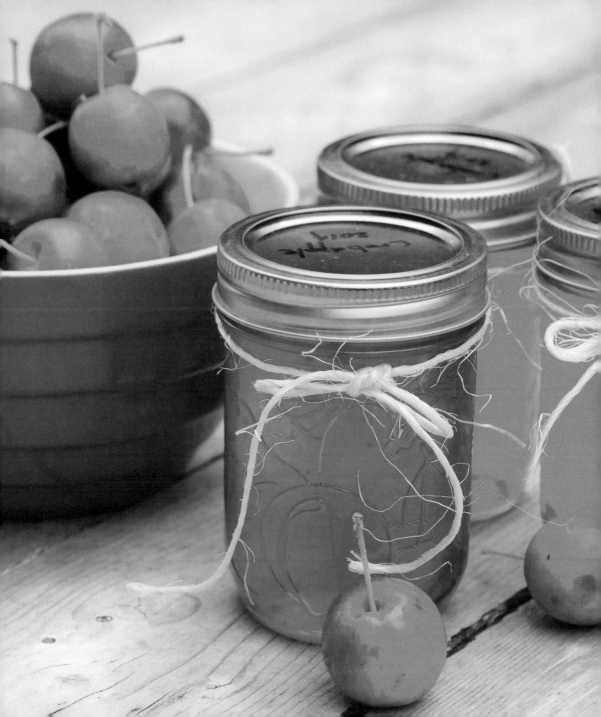

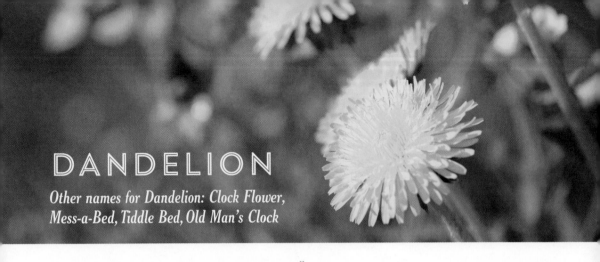

DANDELION

Other names for Dandelion: Clock Flower, Mess-a-Bed, Tiddle Bed, Old Man's Clock

HOW TO IDENTIFY: Probably the most familiar of our wild flowers as it grows everywhere. The beautiful golden yellow flowers shine like little suns in the spring before turning to fluffy dandelion clocks later on in the summer.

The leaves are very distinctive with "Lion's Teeth" (the French being "*dent-du-lion*") edges. The stem is smooth and hollow and will ooze a milky sap once broken open.

HISTORY: It is regarded as a nuisance nowadays by many keen gardeners, but not so long ago it was possible to make a decent living from digging up the roots for use in medicine. As recently as the 1930s, teams of "root diggers" would benefit local farmers by ridding their fields of dandelions. These roots were so sought after for their medicinal properties that a special "green herb" rate was charged for sending them by train to London. A root digger could earn as much as 3d (3 pence) per pound (454 g) in weight for washed roots and 1d (1 penny) per pound in weight for unwashed roots.

Dandelion roots were dried and ground coarsely to be used as a coffee substitute during the rationing of World War II.

FOLKLORE: The childhood joy of gently blowing the seeds off a dandelion globe can not only help you to tell the time, but also tell you how much you are loved. Blow off all the seeds in one go and you are loved with a passion; however, if some seeds remain your partner has some doubts, if lots of seeds remain it might be best to look elsewhere for love.

Blow the seeds in the direction of an absent love to send a message to them.

To give yourself the best chance to all of these superstitions I recommend that you choose a sunny day and a really dry ripe seed head.

If all that wasn't enough, the dandelion globe can also predict the weather. In fine sunny weather the globe is round and fluffy, if rain is on its way the globe shuts like an umbrella until the risk of rain has passed.

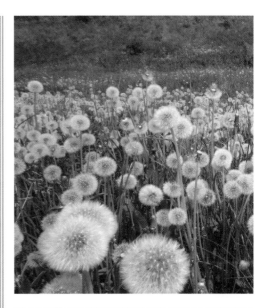

FOLK MEDICINE: An important and commonly used spring tonic, dandelion was regarded as a very powerful cure for many ailments including jaundice and kidney complaints. So effective were dandelion's diuretic properties that children were warned not to touch it or pick it as they would certainly wet the bed that night.

The milky sap from the dandelion stem was rubbed onto warts and allowed to dry; this was repeated until the wart shrivelled away.

OTHER COMMON USES: Dandelion is high in potassium and vitamins A, B, C and D, which can cleanse the blood and stimulate the liver. Young, tender leaves can be mixed into a green salad or made into pesto with pine nuts, olive oil and parmesan cheese. The flowers are traditionally made into wine, beer, cordials, and vodka and, of course, the root combined with burdock root makes a delicious tonic.

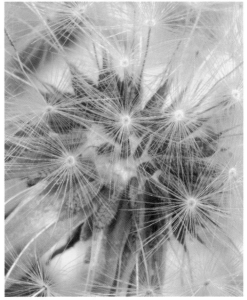

DANDELION FLOWER MUSCLE RUB

A naturally soothing oil to massage into stiff necks and sore muscles. Pick your dandelion flowers on a dry day, away from busy roads and dog walkers.

INGREDIENTS

Enough dandelion flower heads to fill a clean, dry jam jar

Carrier oil of your choice. I like to use peach kernel oil but almond oil or even olive oil will work well too

METHOD

Fill your jam jar with the flower heads.

Slowly pour in your oil making sure that it fills all the gaps between the flowers and there are no bubbles of air.

Cover with a piece of cotton cloth secured with string and place on a sunny windowsill for two weeks or until the oil has turned golden yellow.

Strain, making sure that you squeeze every last drop of oil out of the flowers.

Pour into a clean, dry bottle and use as often as needed.

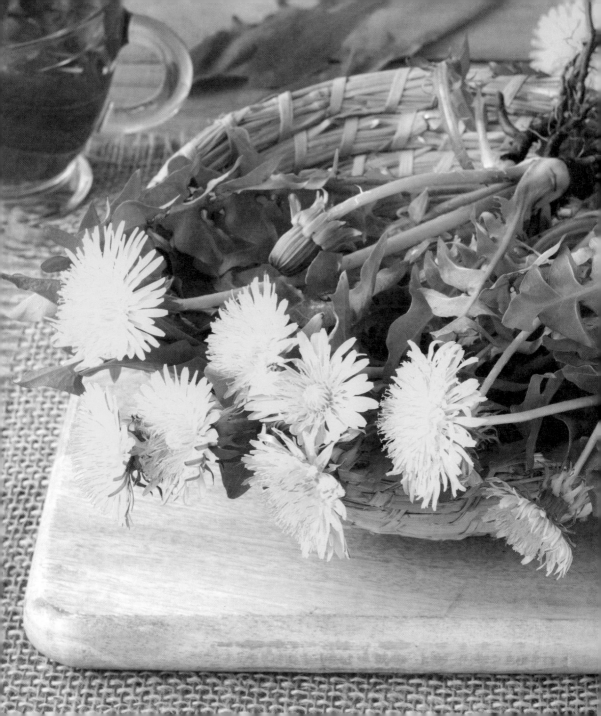

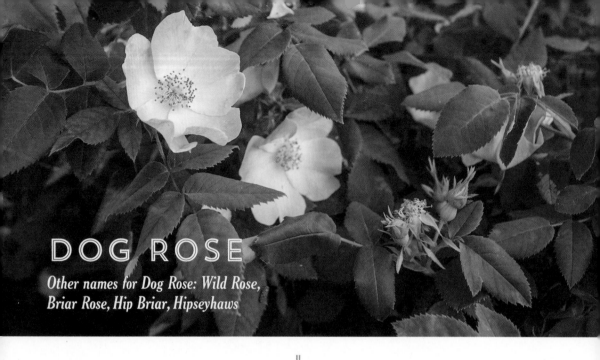

DOG ROSE

Other names for Dog Rose: Wild Rose, Briar Rose, Hip Briar, Hipseyhaws

HOW TO IDENTIFY: A distinctive rambling, sturdy shrub that scrambles through country hedgerows. The tall, arching stems are covered in curved thorns with dark-green, oval-toothed leaves. It produces delicate five-petalled flowers in pink or white from June to July, followed by bright red hips, which light up the autumn hedgerows.

HISTORY: Rosehips contain forty times more vitamin C than oranges do, as well as vitamins A, B and K. During World War II, when citrus fruits were in short supply, rosehips were an important dietary supplement for British children.

Women's institutes, schools, brownies and cubs groups were tasked with going out into the hedgerows to collect this precious hip. It was considered to be your "patriotic duty" to gather rosehips and, by the end of the war, over 2,000 tons had been collected to be made into syrup. Del Rosa paid 3d (3 pence) for every pound (454 g) in weight of rosehips collected, which they then made into syrup to be distributed to children's clinics all over the country. It was to be given to prevent scurvy and other related vitamin C deficiency conditions common in infants at the time.

The fine hairs that are found inside the hips have been used for centuries by mischievous children as "itchy seeds" to be pushed down the jumper of a poor victim. (We've all done it!)

FOLKLORE: Folklore tells us that if we carry rosehips in our pockets we will be protected from getting piles. Schoolboys also carried rosehips in the belief that this would prevent them from getting the cane. Goats with indigestion were fed young shoots of the dog rose, though how you know if a goat has indigestion is a puzzle to me!

Faeries, who wish to become invisible, will eat a rosehip and turn three times widdershins (anti-clockwise). To reappear, they eat another rosehip and turn three times sunwise (clockwise).

FOLK MEDICINE: In traditional folk medicine, rosehips have been used as cure for constipation due to their mild laxative effects.

Dog rose leaves were boiled together with chickweed and the liquid used on sore eyes.

Insects sometimes burrow into the rosehips causing "moss galls"; these were hung inside the house to cure a child of whooping cough. Moss galls were also used to treat insomnia by placing them under the sufferer's pillow, but they must be removed in the morning or the patient might not wake up.

OTHER COMMON USES: The delicate petals of the dog rose can be crystallized by painting them with beaten egg white and then dipping them in sugar to make beautiful edible cake decorations.

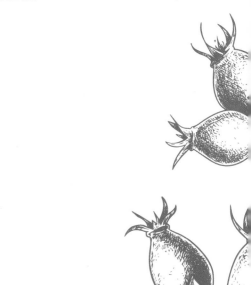

WARTIME ROSEHIP SYRUP

There is a very good reason why old remedies are sometimes the best: many of them actually do work. Although some of the vitamin C is lost during the cooking of this syrup, it is still worth making and using it as a precaution against colds in the autumn months. It tastes pretty good too. Wear long sleeves and gloves to protect yourself from sharp thorns while collecting ripe rosehips from the hedgerows.

Makes around 1.5 litres.

INGREDIENTS

1 kg of ripe rosehips, washed and picked over to remove any dead leaves and suchlike

600 g caster sugar, approximately

1.25 litres of water

METHOD

Roughly chop rosehips using a knife or a food processor.

Bring 1.25 litres of water to the boil in a large pan. Add the chopped rosehips carefully to the boiling water and simmer for 15 minutes, stirring occasionally.

Take off the heat, pop on a lid and leave for 30 minutes.

Allow to drip through a jelly bag or muslin, ensuring that the seeds and hairs don't get into the juice.

Measure the rosehip juice into a saucepan: for every 500 ml of liquid add 300 g of sugar. Heat gently, stirring to dissolve the sugar, and bring to the boil for 3 minutes, skimming off any scum.

Allow to cool slightly, then pour into the prepared bottles and seal tightly. Refrigerate once opened. Use within four months.

A spoonful taken neat every day throughout winter will help to ward off coughs and colds. Also delicious poured over porridge, pancakes and ice cream.

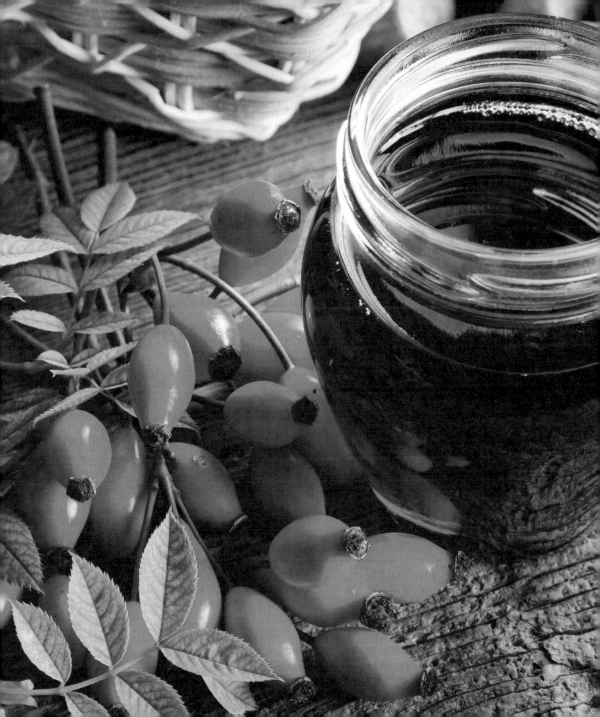

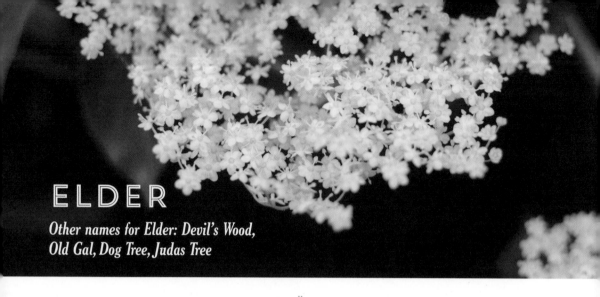

ELDER

Other names for Elder: Devil's Wood,
Old Gal, Dog Tree, Judas Tree

HOW TO IDENTIFY: Common in hedgerows and woods, this small tree has a corky bark that splits as it matures. The leaves are comprised of five to seven oval leaflets with feathery edges. Clusters of creamy white, fragrant flowers appear in summer followed by small purple/black berries in the autumn.

HISTORY: The hollow stems were used like bellows by blacksmiths to blow air onto a fire and young boys once enjoyed using them as peashooters. Elder leaves have insect repelling properties and were often hung from horses' bridles to keep flies away.

FOLKLORE: If you happen to be underneath an elder tree on Midsummer's Night, you may be serenaded by the faery folk playing whistles and pipes made from the hollow stems of the tree. An elder tree that has seeded itself in your garden is said to prevent evil spirits, negative influences and lightning from entering the home, also one planted by a cowshed will protect your cattle.

Elders were believed to be inhabited by witches who had transformed themselves into the tree in order to escape capture. You must always seek permission from the resident witch before you forage from her tree or suffer the consequences.

You risk becoming bewitched if you burn an elder tree in your hearth, the devil will be sitting on the chimney waiting for an opportunity to come in.

According to the *Wiccan Rede*, which was written in the twentieth century as a moral guide for wiccans to abide by:

*"Elder is the lady's tree,
Burn it not or cursed you'll be."*

FOLK MEDICINE: Known by country folk as "nature's medicine chest", every part of this wonderful tree was used as a remedy.

Toothache caused by evil spirits could be cured by chewing on a twig, which was then put on a wall while saying:

"Depart thou evil spirit"

Culpeper also used elder for toothache:

"Take the inner rind of an elder tree, and bruise it, and put thereto a little pepper, and make it into balls, and hold them between the teeth that ache."

Warts could be transferred onto the elder by cutting the same number of notches as you had warts into a piece of root or twig and then rubbing it onto the warts and burying it. As it rots, your warts will vanish.

Scalds and burns were treated with elder flowers mixed with lard to make an ointment. The flowers can also be infused with honey to make tea to soothe the symptoms of hay fever.

An ointment made from the leaves helps to heal bruises, soothe eczema and keep insects away.

The berries are full of antioxidants and vitamin C and were, and still are, used to make an effective home remedy for coughs, colds and sore throats.

OTHER COMMON USES: An English summer wouldn't be the same without a fragrant glass of elderflower cordial in the sunshine. The cordial can also be drizzled over cakes and pancakes and makes a gin and tonic very special indeed!

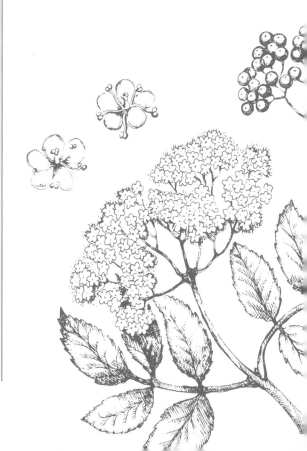

ELDERBERRY ROB

With their wonderful antiviral and antioxidant properties, it's worth freezing elderberries so you can whip up a batch of this medicinal rob any time of year to speed up recovery from coughs, colds and sore throats. The addition of cloves not only helps to preserve the rob, but also lends it their beneficial antiviral and antibacterial properties. Drinking this hot is very soothing. Add a little rum or brandy and a squeeze of lemon for a medicinal hot toddy. Be fussy when you pick elderberries as shrivelled berries won't give up much juice. Pick away from busy roadways and always leave plenty for the birds.

Makes one 750 ml bottle.

INGREDIENTS

500 g ripe elderberries – either fresh or frozen – you can leave them on the stalk

Water

10 whole cloves, approximately

300 g caster sugar, approximately

Sterilized bottles

METHOD

Place your berries in a large pan. Ensure it is large enough not to boil over. Add water until the berries are just floating.

Slowly bring to the boil and simmer for 15 minutes.

Use a potato masher to burst any berries that are still whole.

Carefully pour the liquid through a colander and into a large jug, using the masher to squeeze out as much juice as you can. It's worth taking time to do this as the best juice comes out right at the end.

Pour the liquid through a sieve and measure your juice into a pan. For every 500 ml of juice, add 300 g of sugar and ten cloves.

Bring slowly to the boil, stirring constantly to dissolve the sugar.

Boil hard for 5 minutes, then allow to cool slightly before pouring into sterile bottles and labelling.

This rob can be taken neat or diluted with hot water.

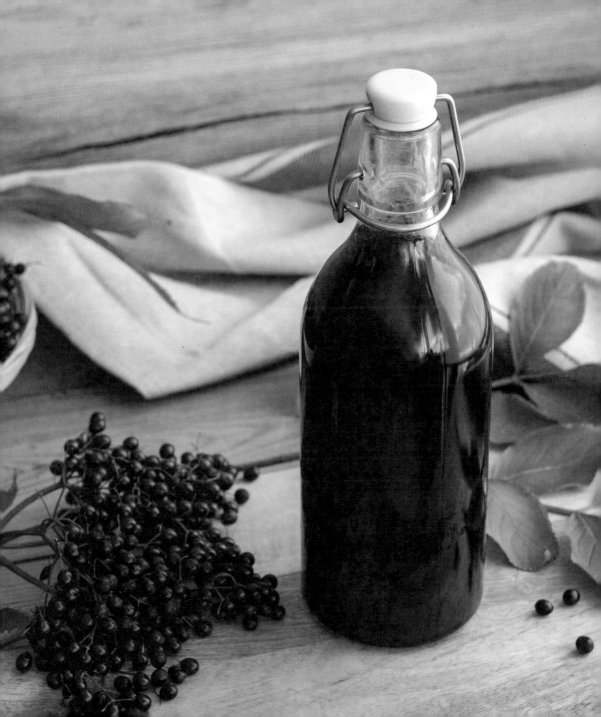

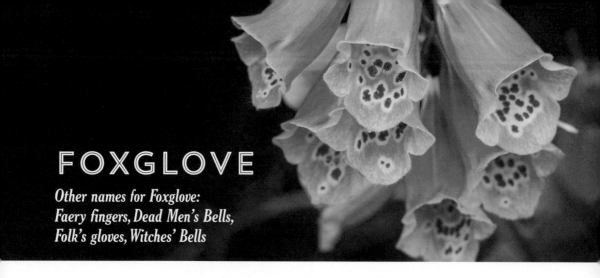

FOXGLOVE

Other names for Foxglove:
Faery fingers, Dead Men's Bells,
Folk's gloves, Witches' Bells

HOW TO IDENTIFY: The foxglove is easily identifiable once in flower but beware – all parts of this plant are potentially poisonous to humans and some animals. Always wear gloves when handling foxgloves and NEVER ingest any part of the plant.

Foxgloves prefer shady woodland, verges and, of course, cottage gardens. They have large flat leaves at the base followed by majestic tall spikes of bell-shaped purple flowers in early summer that open from the bottom up.

HISTORY: In the eighteenth century, a young country doctor, William Withering, grew frustrated watching potential patients visit the local wise woman instead of coming to him. He tried to discredit her by spreading rumours that she was a witch, but her patients were loyal. He saw a man,

who he knew to have heart problems, pay a visit to the wise woman. He then observed her picking foxglove leaves in her garden with which to treat the man. He never did make a success of his country practice, but he went on to write *An Account of the Foxglove and some of its Medicinal Uses*, which led to further research and the drug digoxin being developed.

FOLKLORE: As with bluebells, the distinctive bell shape of the foxglove has always been associated with faery folklore. Here is one medieval ritual using foxgloves that is definitely not recommended. Badly behaved or surly children were often labelled "changelings", meaning that parents believed their innocent children had been swapped for a faery child. There was a sure-fire test to determine whether or not your child was a changeling: three drops of foxglove juice were placed on the child's tongue and three drops in each ear, they were then made to sit on a shovel which was swung three times through an open doorway saying:

"If you're a fairy, away with you."

In Scotland, foxglove leaves were put into babies' cradles to protect them from evil. The connection between foxgloves and children seems to be a common theme, naughty children who knew that faeries hid inside the flowers would strike the flower bell hoping to hear "faery thunder" as the annoyed creature made her escape.

Tall foxgloves bend and sway elegantly, not because of the breeze, but because they bow down with respect when they recognize faeries and other mystical beings passing by.

Planting foxgloves in your garden will encourage faeries to live there and hopefully keep evil away. If this doesn't work, black dye made from the leaves can be painted onto your cottage floor in the shape of a cross for protection.

Foxes wear the little bell-shaped slippers on their paws, enabling them to sneak into the chicken coop at night without being heard – hence the name!

FOLK MEDICINE: Foxglove was used to treat a number of ailments from a poultice for bad knees to eczema in animals. A handwritten note, now held in a Scottish museum and believed to date from the early nineteenth century, gives us an insight into one of the remedies:

"For a man in great pain from an internal growth or swelling, a pulp was made from squashed foxglove roots, then applied inside flannel, after the pulp had been heated, as a poultice to the swelling. The man received immediate relief, and continued to do so until the cure was completed."

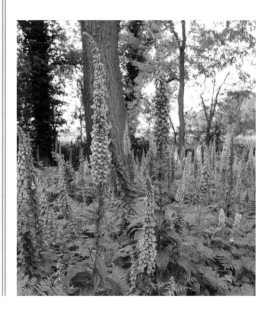

ITCHY WITCH STICK

Foxgloves, along with many other common plants, can cause skin irritation and, as a forager, you will always attract annoying insect bites and nettle stings. Please be aware of the potentially toxic nature of foxgloves, wash hands after contact or, better still, always wear gloves. Although we can't use foxgloves in our remedy here, the foxglove is still an incredibly beautiful plant that can be much admired and photographed while out enjoying the countryside.

Made with soothing witch hazel, anti-inflammatory lavender, and peppermint to cool and relieve itching and to repel insects, I like to put this handy remedy into a small roller-ball bottle to carry with me whenever I'm out in the countryside.

Makes 100 ml.

INGREDIENTS

90 ml witch hazel

10 ml glycerin (this keeps the oils in suspension)

10 drops lavender essential oil

10 drops lemon essential oil

6 drops peppermint essential oil

METHOD

Mix all ingredients in a clean jug.

Pour into a dark bottle or small roller ball bottles (available online).

Shake before use, keeps for about one year.

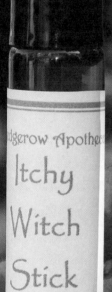

Hedgerow Apothec...

Itchy
Witch
Stick

...f for bites and sting...

...hazel, Glycerine, Laver...
...permint & Lemon E. Oil...

Hedgerow Apoth...

Itchy
Witch
Stick

...ef for bites and s...

...ch hazel, Glycerine, La...
...Peppermint & Lemon E...

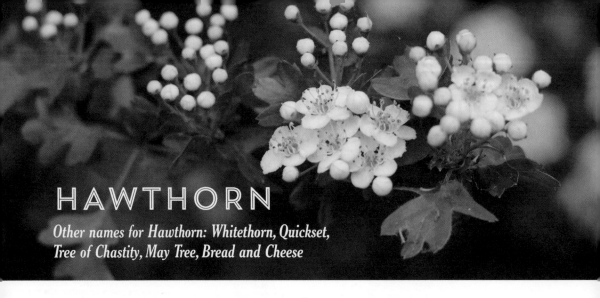

HAWTHORN

*Other names for Hawthorn: Whitethorn, Quickset,
Tree of Chastity, May Tree, Bread and Cheese*

HOW TO IDENTIFY: Found growing in most hedgerows, the hawthorn has small, deep-lobed leaves that look almost divided. Young stems are reddish in colour with sharp thorns, hence the name. In spring it is covered in an abundance of delicate white flowers known as "May blossom" and these turn into dark, berry-like fruits known as "haws" in the autumn.

HISTORY: During her Kentish childhood in the 1940s, my mother-in-law tells me that she often picked the leaves and buds of the hawthorn tree to eat as a snack on the way to and from school. This was known as "bread and cheese" and has a nutty, pleasant taste as long as it's eaten young in early spring before the flowers are in full bloom.

One of Britain's ancient and most common trees, prickly hawthorn was planted to enclose fields as its dense coverage would keep livestock from wandering.

The first pilgrims to America named their ship *The Mayflower* as hawthorn wood was used to make some pieces of the vessel.

During World War I, young hawthorn leaves were used as a substitute for both tea and tobacco, and the seeds were ground and used instead of coffee.

FOLKLORE: Even into the twentieth century, at calving and lambing time, the afterbirth would be thrown on top of a hawthorn hedge to ensure the fertility of the next generation of animals.

This old English nursery rhyme reminds young ladies that they need to get up very early on May Day to take advantage of this beneficial piece of folklore:

"The fair maid who, the first of May,
goes to the fields at break of day,
And washes in the dew from the hawthorn
tree, will ever after handsome be."

It is said that a twig of hawthorn, tied together with twigs from an oak tree and an ash tree using red thread, will provide protection from faeries.

During the country custom of "going a-Maying", branches would be cut and woven to adorn doorways and windows (although hawthorn rarely flowers on May Day). The weaving was important because it strengthened the plant's magical powers, as did its exposure to the overnight dew. Using the blossoms for decorations outside was allowed, but superstitious people believed that hawthorn flowers should never be brought into the house as death is sure to follow, possibly because of the putrid smell of hawthorn flowers.

FOLK MEDICINE: An infusion of the flowers and leaves was used to treat sore throats, while chewing the bark gave relief from toothache. Unfortunate slugs would, once again, be impaled on the hawthorn spikes in an effort to cure warts.

In the nineteenth century, it was discovered that haws were very useful in treating heart conditions, as well as normalizing blood pressure.

OTHER COMMON USES: Adding haws to other hedgerow fruit makes a delicious fruity jelly.

Modern medicine has recognized its considerable benefits to heart health. It has been found to lower blood pressure, open the arteries and strengthen the heart.

It is important not to take hawthorn if you use beta-blockers and other heart drugs without the advice of a qualified medical practitioner.

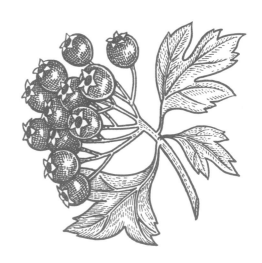

HEDGEROW JELLY

All of these hedgerow fruits are full of vitamins, minerals and fibre. I always use less sugar than traditional recipes recommend, this means that your jelly will not keep for quite as long but, believe me, you'll love being able to taste the delicious fruit and not just the sugar.

Makes three to four 500 g jars.

INGREDIENTS

1 kg of foraged crab apples or cooking apples, washed and cut into chunks, including pips and core

1 kg mixed hedgerow fruit: haws, blackberries, sloes, chopped rosehips

Water

750 g white sugar, approximately

METHOD

Put all your fruit into a large pan and add just enough water to make it float.

Bring to a simmer for about 30 minutes – until all the fruit is cooked and pulpy. Tip into a jelly bag or muslin and allow the juice to drip into a bowl overnight.

Measure the juice, and for every 600 ml, add 450 g of sugar.

Bring slowly to the boil, stirring to dissolve the sugar. Bring to a rolling boil for 5–10 minutes, until setting point has been reached.

Check for setting point using the wrinkle test. Before you begin, put a couple of small plates into the freezer. Bring your jelly to the boil as above, take the pan off the heat and carefully put a little jelly onto one of the cold plates. Let it stand for a minute, then push the blob with your finger; you should see it wrinkle. If the jelly is still liquid, pop it back on the heat for another 5 minutes and then test again.

Pour into hot, sterilized jars with screw top lids and label them.

Keep in the fridge once open. Use within one year.

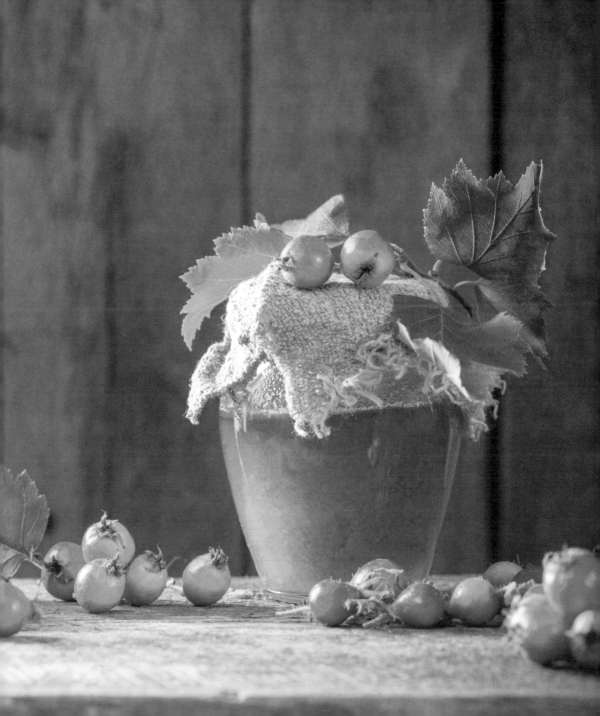

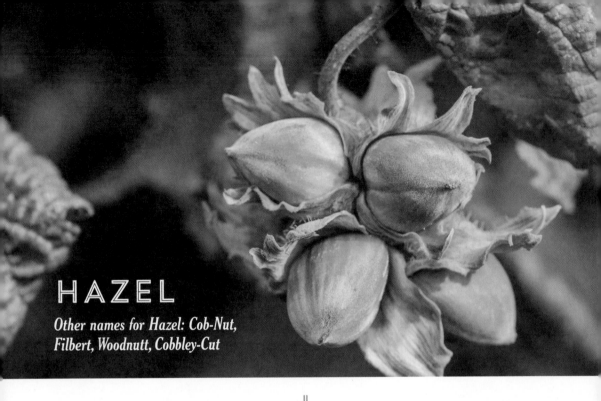

HAZEL

Other names for Hazel: Cob-Nut, Filbert, Woodnutt, Cobbley-Cut

HOW TO IDENTIFY: Hazel is abundant in the UK. It typically grows to between 3–8 metres (10–26 feet) tall, and can be found in hedgerows and woods. The tooth-edged leaves appear in early May and are often tinged with red, with deep lines running down their length. Flowers appear in autumn and can be open as early as January. The male flower is a long yellow catkin and the female flower is much smaller and bud-like. The female flowers are the ones that develop into delicious hazelnuts, which ripen in late summer and are much coveted by squirrels, mice and people.

HISTORY: On Holy Cross Day, which fell on 14 September 629 BC, a piece of the true Christian cross was thought to have been recovered and stored in Constantinople. In 1560, Eton schoolboys were given a half-day off school to commemorate Holy Cross Day and they decided to have some fun by gathering nuts to eat and so the tradition of "nutting" was born. Up until the early 1900s, schoolchildren were given the day off school on Holy Cross Day, simply so they could go "nutting" with their families.

Early man used the hazel's flexible properties to make baskets and to construct wattle walls, and there is evidence that hazel was grown and coppiced hundreds of years ago.

FOLKLORE: May Day is the traditional time to collect hazel wood as this is when it is at its most powerful to use for protection. Hazel fences were built around dwellings because it was impossible for evil to penetrate them. On May Day, malevolent faeries were known to abduct children and babies and sneak into the dairy to curdle the milk in the dead of night. An amulet made from hazel wood was worn as protection against these mischievous creatures.

Catkins were brought into the house at lambing time to safeguard the expectant ewes, and small bundles of twigs were used to shield the home from thunder and lightning. If you wish your baby's eyes to be brown in colour, slip some hazel twigs into the infant's room.

Hazel catkins have long been associated with childbirth and fertility, and there were many traditional sayings to demonstrate this, as Gabrielle Hatfield records in her book, *Hatfield's Herbal* (2007):

> *"Plenty of catkins, plenty of prams."*

Another traditional saying regarding the fertility associated with the hazelnuts goes like this:

> *"Many nuts in the autumn, means lots of babies in the spring."*

It was futile to ignore these words of wisdom, as one newly married Somerset girl found out. She publicly announced her intention not to have any children as she valued her freedom. Locals all gave her a present of a large bag of hazelnuts, and four children soon followed.

FOLK MEDICINE: In some parts of Britain, hazelnuts were carried as charms to ward off rheumatism. Two hazelnuts on one stalk is known as a "loady-nut", and as well as protecting you from the "evil eye", it would also cure your toothache. The Celts believed that the hazelnut represented concentrated wisdom and, if that isn't enough, it was even used to forecast the weather:

> *"If the nut shells are thick, the winter will be bleak. If the nut shells are thin the winter will be mild."*

OTHER COMMON USES: Woodland crafts using hazel twigs are ever-popular, as the twigs can be twisted and knotted into many shapes. Wild hazelnuts, often called cobnuts, are still grown in Kent but, alas, most of our hazelnuts are now imported.

HAZELNUT BUTTER

I just love making nut butters! They taste great, are free from the palm oil often included in commercial nut butters, and are rich in magnesium, calcium, unsaturated fats and vitamins B and E. Plus, they are delicious and really easy to make!

Makes approximately one 500 g jar.

INGREDIENTS

400 g blanched hazelnuts or cobnuts

3 tbsp organic cacao powder

2 tbsp maple syrup

½ tsp sea salt

METHOD

Roast your hazelnuts on a baking tray at 180°C (356°F) for about 10 minutes or until golden brown. They burn easily, so keep watch! Allow to cool.

Tip the nuts into a food processor, add the cacao, maple syrup and salt. This is possible with a pestle and mortar but will be very hard work!

Grind for about 5 minutes, stopping to push the mixture down occasionally. At first it will just look like sand, but be patient...

And, as if by magic, it will suddenly turn into a creamy, velvety butter. Keep whizzing until it is completely smooth.

If you feel it is too thick, add a drizzle of hazelnut oil and grind again.

Spoon into a clean, dry jar.

The same recipe works just as well using peanuts.

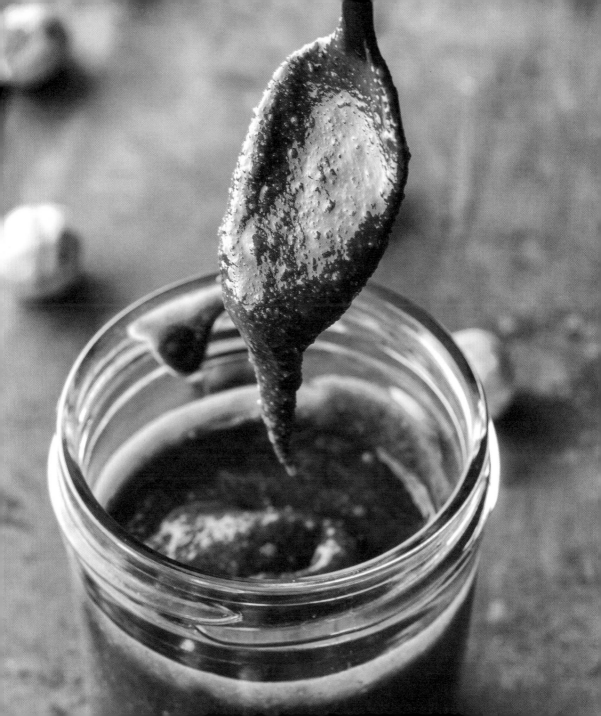

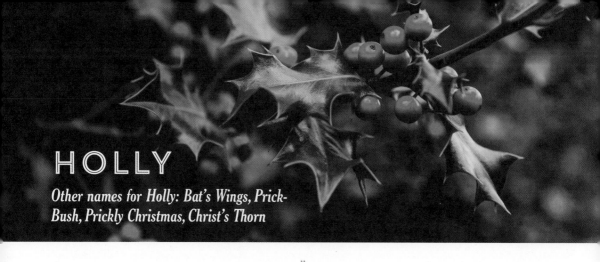

HOLLY

Other names for Holly: Bat's Wings, Prick-Bush, Prickly Christmas, Christ's Thorn

HOW TO IDENTIFY: Holly is very easily identifiable from both images on Christmas cards and holly wreaths. This evergreen shrub can grow to 15 metres (50 feet) tall, and live for 200 years. Leaves are glossy, thick, dark green and usually prickly; they grow alternately on the stems. Once pollinated by insects, the white female flowers turn into the familiar red or orange berries which remain on the tree throughout winter.

HISTORY: Holly was banned as decoration in churches due to its pagan associations, however, in the 1600s, many stories appeared that linked holly to Christian stories. According to legend, the first holly sprung up where Jesus had trodden, and it was considered to be symbolic of His blood and suffering.

Early Christians adopted the Roman festival of Saturnalia, which was celebrated throughout December along with the tradition of sending holly boughs and gifts to friends at this time.

With a reputation for being a very protective plant, hollies were often planted to mark the boundaries of properties and it was considered bad luck to cut them down.

The wood of the holly, which is hard and white, was carved into white chess pieces, ebony being used for the black set. In Royal Tunbridge Wells, Kent, it was used to make the famous intricately decorated Tunbridge ware boxes.

FOLKLORE: There are two types of holly leaf: the prickly leaf, which was regarded as masculine and the smooth leaf, which was regarded as feminine. This fact was important when bringing in the holly for Christmas: if the smooth holly was brought in first, the woman of the household would be master for the following year, if the prickly holly came in first, then the man would rule.

Holly has long been believed to have protective powers. It was said to protect a house from lightning and, if given to newlyweds, it would keep the couple safe from evil influences.

In medieval England, unmarried women would tie a sprig of holly or ivy to their beds to protect them from ghosts and evil spirits in winter time. It was believed that supernatural creatures were more active during Christmastime due to the piercing winter winds and the creaks caused by wild storms. Since the holly and the ivy were protectors of women who followed the pagan religion, they were forbidden to appear inside the Christian home. For this reason, it was used in the form of a wreath to decorate the outside of the home, still serving to protect the occupants from evil spirits. The wreath is traditionally circular, associated with the eternal cycle of nature, the changing seasons and fertility in paganism, and adopted in Christianity to signify that Christ has no beginning and no end and representing everlasting life.

Before the Victorians introduced Christmas trees into homes, great spheres of holly decorated with fruit and ribbons were brought in. Some included mistletoe and were called "kissing balls".

FOLK MEDICINE: In the nineteenth and early twentieth century, chilblains were cured by thrashing them with spiky holly leaves or sometimes rubbing an ointment made from powdered holly berries onto the sores.

A cup made from the wood of a holly tree was given to children to drink from when they had whooping cough. Rather disturbingly, if they had worms, the children would yawn over a bowl containing water with holly and sage and the worm was believed to drop out.

OTHER COMMON USES: Holly hedges and trees provide vital food and shelter for our native birds through winter.

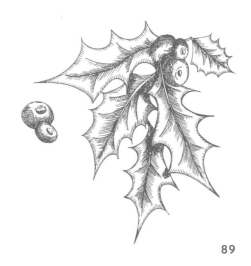

SKELETON LEAVES

Skeleton leaves are so beautiful, delicate and lacy. They can be used to decorate Christmas cards and photo albums. Children can have fun with this craft too.

INGREDIENTS

1 tbsp baking powder

1 tbsp bicarbonate of soda

1 litre of cold water

Fresh leaves

An old toothbrush

METHOD

Dissolve the baking powder and bicarbonate of soda in a saucepan containing cold water.

Put your leaves into the pan, slowly bring to the boil and simmer while stirring occasionally. The water will become murky and brown and froth up. Don't worry, this is fine.

After about half an hour, the leaves should be ready.

Take one leaf out of the pan at a time and put it into a shallow tray of clean water. Using the old toothbrush, gently clean away the leaf pulp to reveal the skeleton.

Carefully place the skeleton leaves onto a paper towel to dry.

Use the skeleton leaves as decoration for all sorts of craft projects.

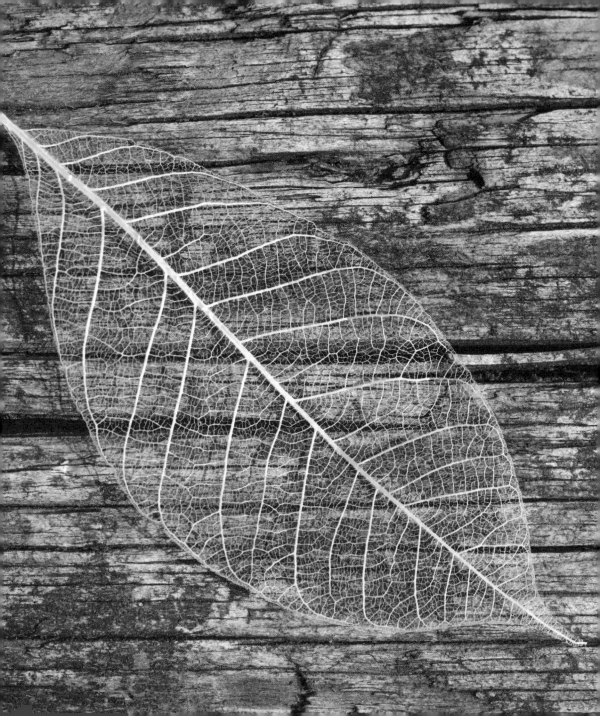

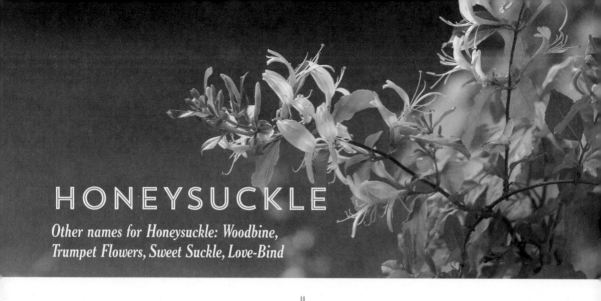

HONEYSUCKLE

Other names for Honeysuckle: Woodbine, Trumpet Flowers, Sweet Suckle, Love-Bind

HOW TO IDENTIFY: Smaller than the cultivated garden variety, the wild honeysuckle twirls its way up hedgerows and trees creating a heady, sweet scent that is carried on the breeze. Distinctive yellowy-white, trumpet-like flowers appear in summer, attracting pollinators at dusk when their scent is at its most fragrant. Clusters of red berries ripen in the autumn to be gratefully devoured by warblers, thrushes and bullfinches.

HISTORY: Countless children over the years have enjoyed sucking the sweet-tasting nectar from the base of the trumpet-shaped flowers, hence the name "honeysuckle". England's woodland was far more abundant during the time of William Shakespeare than it is now, and Shakespeare would have seen honeysuckle growing wild everywhere. He mentions honeysuckle in several of his plays. Titania to Bottom in *A Midsummer Night's Dream*:

> *"Sleep though, and I will*
> *wind thee in my arms...*
> *So doth the woodbine,*
> *the sweet honeysuckle,*
> *Gently entwist."*

And,

> *"I know a bank where*
> *the wild thyme blows,*
> *Where oxlips grow and*
> *violets nod their heads,*
> *Canopied with luscious*
> *honeysuckle..."*

When honeysuckle grows, it winds itself tightly around the host tree, sometimes causing spiralling grooves. Hazel sticks that were misshapen in this way were known in Sussex as "honeysuckle sticks" and were used as walking sticks with the added bonus that they were thought to attract luck, especially with the ladies.

FOLKLORE: Honeysuckle is a good plant to grow around your doorway; it will bring wealth and protect the family from illness and black magic as well as being attractive and fragrant.

Opinion seems to vary from region to region as to whether it is a good idea to bring honeysuckle into the house. It was considered unlucky to bring it inside in Wales, but in Somerset, its intertwining stems would encourage marriage and even promote erotic dreams if placed in the bedroom. Gently crushing fresh flowers on the forehead were said to heighten your psychic powers.

FOLK MEDICINE: Culpeper holds honeysuckle in high regard as he:

"Knows no better cure for asthma."

An infusion of honeysuckle flowers was used to treat asthma and other lung complaints.

The leaves are rich in salicylic acid, a component of aspirin, which makes them an effective treatment for headaches, flu, colds and general aches and pains.

A poultice of dried honeysuckle was placed onto warts to heal them, far nicer than some of the other cures for warts that were fashionable at the time!

OTHER COMMON USES: The flowers can be used in teas, jellies, jams, for making country wine and decorating cakes.

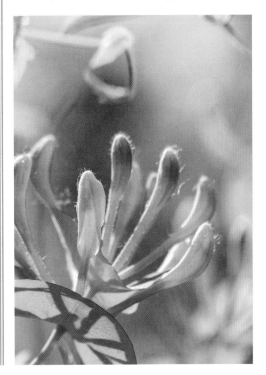

HONEYSUCKLE HONEY FOR SORE THROATS

Honeysuckle flowers are still used today to treat coughs, sore throats, bronchitis and flu. Make some of this delicious remedy when the flowers are at their best to keep for when those inevitable winter "nasties" come along. Honeysuckle honey can also be rubbed onto chicken pox to speed up healing (always do a patch test first).

INGREDIENTS

Fresh honeysuckle flowers

Clean jar with lid

1 jar of good-quality, local, raw, runny honey

METHOD

Fill the jar with honeysuckle flowers and buds, gently packing them down as you go. Pour in the runny honey, stirring to make sure that all the flowers are submerged (if they pop out, they may go bad).

Allow to settle and top up with more honey if necessary.

Place in a cool, dark place for about four weeks to allow the honeysuckle to infuse.

Strain out the flowers. You may have to gently warm the honey to do this, but do not boil as all the good, healing bacteria will be destroyed over 40°C (104°F).

Take a spoonful as often as needed.

Use within one year.

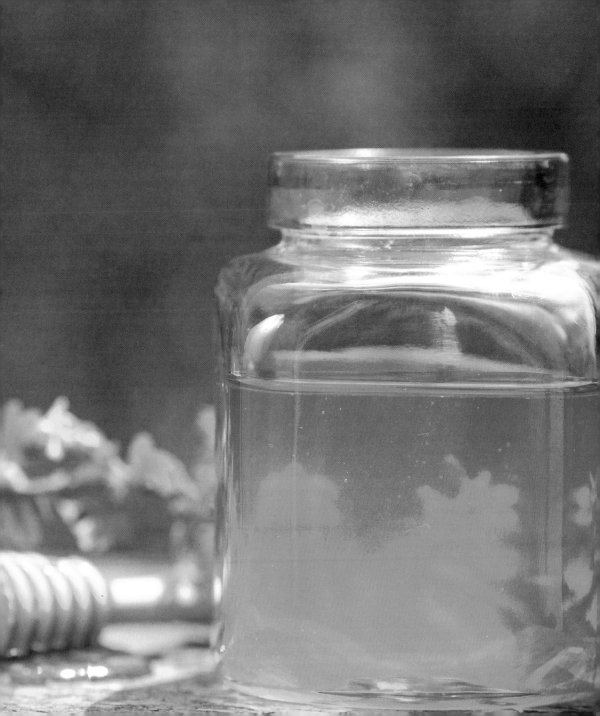

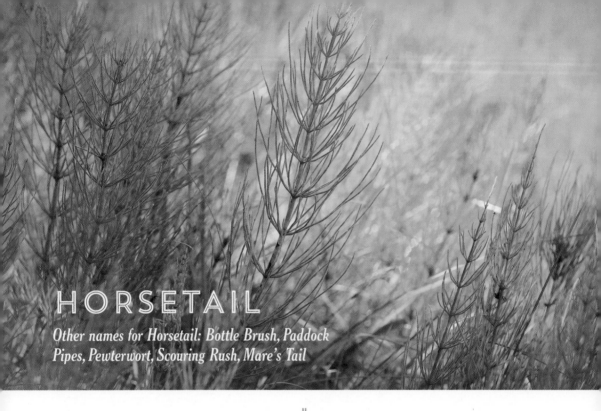

HORSETAIL

Other names for Horsetail: Bottle Brush, Paddock Pipes, Pewterwort, Scouring Rush, Mare's Tail

HOW TO IDENTIFY: Deep in the ground, horsetail rhizomes wait for spring before showing their parasol-shaped stems above ground. Commonly found on waste ground, railway embankments and fields, the bristled stems grow to around 80 cm (30 inches) tall. It does not have hairs or leaves; the bristles are formed by thin, barren stems. Horsetail doesn't flower; it reproduces in the same way as ferns, with spores that are produced in the cone-shaped clusters of small green branches. These tufty green branches produce quite a haze of green foliage and the plant closely resembles a bottle brush.

HISTORY: This is one of our oldest native plants with examples of horsetail having been found in fossils from over 350 million years ago. Horsetail is the main source of silica in the plant kingdom; silica is a mineral vital for the structure and strength of bones and joints, keeps skin supple, makes hair shiny and fingernails strong.

The stem contains so much abrasive silica that it was often used to polish metals, as a light sandpaper, to clean wooden kitchen utensils and to scour milk pails. The plant was sold on the streets of London as a cleaning agent up until the eighteenth century, and it was said that powdered horsetail ash mixed with water was by far the best way to polish silver.

FOLKLORE: Placing horsetail in the bedrooms of couples who are struggling to conceive is supposed to increase the fertility of those who sleep there; adding it to drinks is said to have the same effect. The stems of the horsetail plant are hollow and have been used to make whistles that are thought to attract snakes – why anyone would want to do that is a mystery to me!

FOLK MEDICINE: Culpeper often used horsetail to help staunch bleeding:

> *"It is very powerful to stop bleeding either inward or outward, the juice of the decoction being drunk, or the juice, decoction or distilled water applied outwardly."*

The ashes of the plant, as well as being an excellent silver polish as mentioned above, were also used to treat stomach acid and indigestion *and "an infusion of the dried herb is frequently used as a tea for poor people with diarrhoea"*.

OTHER COMMON USES: In modern herbal medicine, horsetail is used for fluid retention, kidney and bladder stones and urine infections as well as osteoporosis. It can improve brittle fingernails and help with the production of collagen for healthy skin and shiny hair.

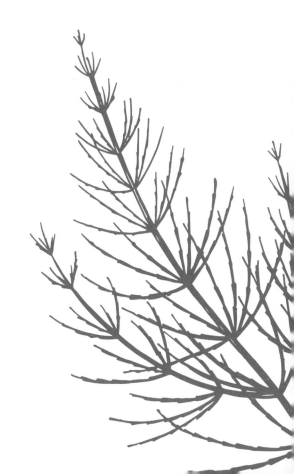

HEALTHY HAIR MIST

Utilizing the natural properties of herbs and essential oils, this hair mist will stimulate growth and encourage shiny, healthy hair. Horsetail is high in silica for strength and shine; nettle is rich in iron and vitamins A, C and K, plus magnesium and potassium to help stimulate hair growth; aloe vera gel naturally soothes the scalp and makes the mist silky smooth; and essential oils of rosemary, lavender and clary sage are all known to promote skin and hair health.

Makes 300 ml of solution.

INGREDIENTS

2 tbsp dried horsetail

2 tbsp dried nettle leaf

250 ml natural spring water

300 ml spray bottle

2 tbsp organic aloe vera gel

10 drops rosemary essential oil

10 drops lavender essential oil

10 drops clary sage essential oil

METHOD

Place the dried horsetail and nettle leaves into a jug.

Boil the spring water and pour it over them.

Let the herbs infuse until the water becomes cold.

Strain out the herbs and pour the liquid into a spray bottle.

Add the aloe vera and essential oils and shake well.

Spray liberally onto the hair roots once or twice a day.

Shake well before each use. Keeps for about three months if stored in the fridge.

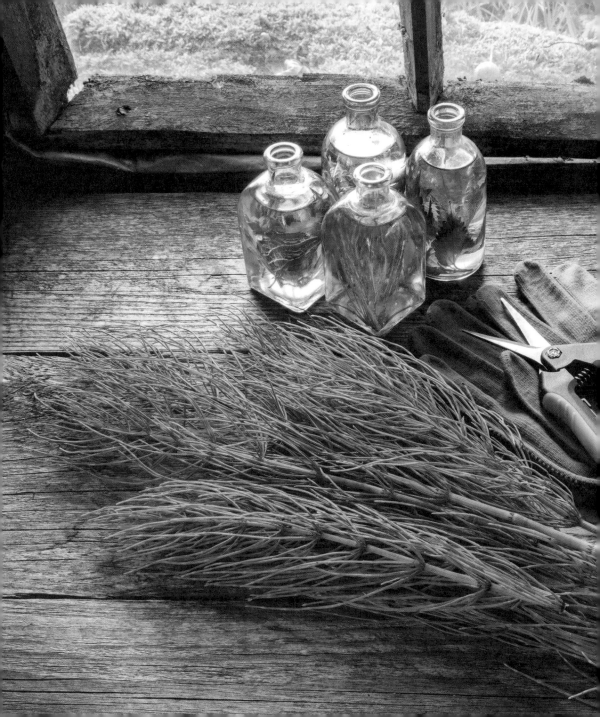

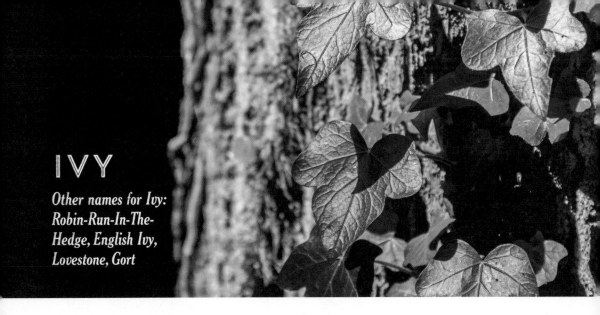

IVY

*Other names for Ivy:
Robin-Run-In-The-
Hedge, English Ivy,
Lovestone, Gort*

HOW TO IDENTIFY: Ivy is an evergreen woody climber, usually seen scrambling up trees and walls. It provides vital food and shelter for our native wildlife, although many gardeners fail to see its importance and believe that it strangles trees. Leaves are glossy and dark green, heart-shaped or oval with pale veins. Flowers are pale yellow umbels and appear between September and November, before turning into black spherical clusters of berries.

HISTORY: Seen as a symbol of achievement, ivy wreaths were presented to winners of poetry competitions in ancient Rome and to champion athletes in ancient Greece.

Ivy was included in bridal bouquets to represent fidelity and good luck, especially for the bride as ivy was regarded as a "feminine" plant. Today it is still the custom for bridal bouquets to contain a sprig of ivy.

Victorian servants boiled ivy leaves in water until it turned black, this was then used to revive the colour of black silk or to remove the shine from fabrics.

FOLKLORE: Wreaths and crowns have been made from ivy for centuries by both our Christian and our non-Christian ancestors. Representing immortality, it was twisted together with bramble and rowan and either worn on the head or placed in the doorways of cowsheds as protection from infection and the "evil eye".

An ivy leaf should be picked on New Year's Eve and placed in a dish of water and covered. Leave it there until the Twelfth Night and then take it out; if the leaf is still green then you will have good health for the following year.

In English folklore, ivy is seen as a kindly plant that is a symbol of friendship and female fertility; it is evergreen even in the depths of a long cold winter. Because of its obvious pagan associations, ivy was banned from houses and churches for many hundreds of years.

FOLK MEDICINE: An ivy wreath worn "with perseverance" is said to prevent hair from thinning. When the moon was waning was the best time to treat corns and warts with an ivy leaf dipped in vinegar. Stems boiled in butter eased sunburn and children drank from cups made from ivy wood in an effort to cure whooping cough.

The preacher John Wesley walked up to 5,000 miles (approximately 8,000 km) a year and was known to rub ivy leaves onto his feet to relieve them of their soreness.

The plague swept through London in 1665 and ivy berries soaked in vinegar were regularly applied to the sores.

The soothing properties of ivy were further illustrated in a twentieth century Cornish parish magazine:

"Gamekeepers whose eyes became inflamed with exposure to gunpowder fumes discovered that they could obtain relief by using an infusion of ground ivy made with boiling water to bathe them. The notion is believed to have originated from itinerant gypsies."

Ivy is the plant dedicated to Bacchus, Roman god of wine and drunkenness, and is often seen on pub signs. A handful of crushed ivy leaves boiled in wine was believed to prevent the drinker from becoming intoxicated and wives who wanted to curb their husbands' habit would spread ivy leaves across the garden path for him to walk over. It was also believed that if an alcoholic drank from a cup made out of ivy wood, they would be cured.

OTHER COMMON USES: Ivy grows quickly and can provide lots of winter cover in the garden, as well as being very beneficial to wildlife. Its pliable stems mean that it can be twisted into swags and wreaths to decorate the home at Christmas.

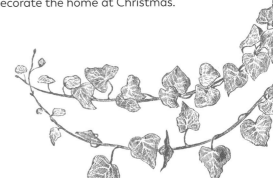

IVY TONING OIL

Ivy contains hederagenin which, along with rosemary essential oil, increases the blood flow to the part of the body it is applied to, and lemon evens out skin tone.

Makes 500 ml of solution.

INGREDIENTS

500 ml organic olive oil

Dark-coloured glass bottle or jar

20 fresh ivy leaves

10 drops of rosemary essential oil

5 drops of lemon essential oil

METHOD

Pour the oil into the dark-coloured bottle or jar, add the ivy leaves and essential oils and shake well.

Place in a warm, dark place such as an airing cupboard.

Shake once a day for 40 days, then strain and bottle.

Rub gently into the hips and thighs every night to help reduce cellulite.

Do not use if allergic to ivy.

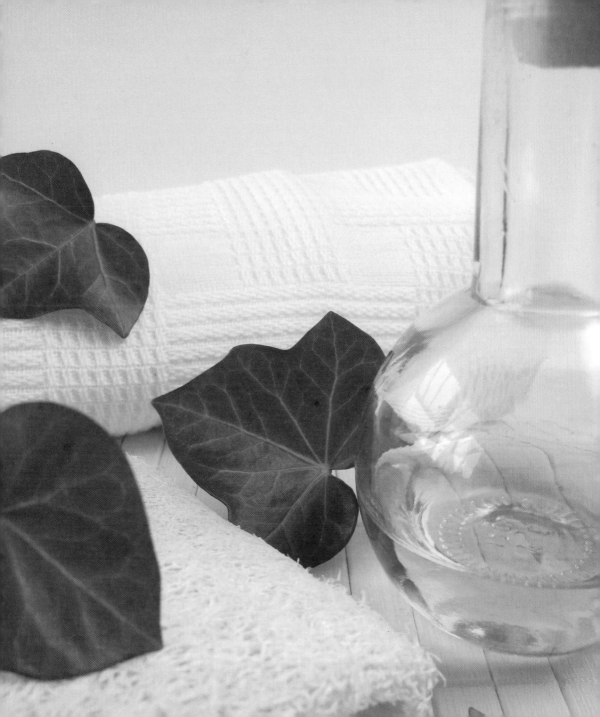

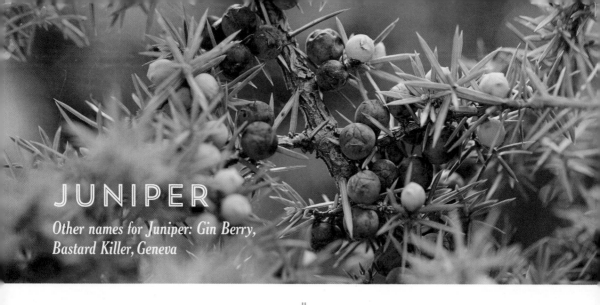

JUNIPER

Other names for Juniper: Gin Berry, Bastard Killer, Geneva

HOW TO IDENTIFY: Juniper is one of the characteristic heathland shrubs of chalk and limestone areas. The leaves take the form of needles and are a deep green colour, sometimes with a bluish tinge. On account of its needle-like leaves, it is often known in folk tradition as the "needle yew". The berries usually take two to three years to ripen fully; it is common to see both the bluish-black ripe berries alongside very green and under-ripe ones on the same bush. When fully ripe, the berries are about the size of a pea and have an aromatic, resiny scent.

HISTORY: There is some evidence that the juniper may have been one of the first shrubs to colonize the British Isles as the ice sheets retreated at the end of the last Ice Age, about 12,000 years ago. Extremely hardy, juniper was able to establish itself on the emerging tundra and its prickles appear to have given it more protection from grazing animals than other less well-protected trees.

Romans used juniper berries as a pungent alternative to the very expensive peppercorns of the time.

Juniper wood burns slowly and doesn't produce much smoke – useful when you have an illicit distilling operation on the go!

FOLKLORE: Despite having a grim history, juniper was regarded as having many beneficial magical powers. A sprig of juniper worn on clothing would give protection from accidents, drive away snakes and demons and break any spells that have been cast against the wearer.

Babies that were teething were regarded to be particularly vulnerable to the influences of supernatural powers and so teething rings were created from juniper in an effort to protect the infant.

Simply carrying the berries was regarded as a strong aphrodisiac and it was often popped into potions in an effort to encourage love, ironic when you consider its medicinal use (see below). In the eighteenth century gin was mainly drunk by poorer members of the population as it was much cheaper than other forms of alcohol at the time. Gin was given to babies to stop them crying and women fell into prostitution to enable them to buy it – leading to it being nicknamed "mother's ruin"!

In the Scottish Highlands on New Year's morning, juniper was burned in the house and byre (cowshed) to purify both buildings and inhabitants. Throughout Europe, there was a custom of burning juniper berries in the house for three days leading up to Beltane (May Day) to fumigate the house and welcome summer. Folk custom in the south west of England states that you should burn juniper wood and needles close to a sick person to vaporize the oils, cleansing the room of the sickness.

FOLK MEDICINE: Juniper was burned during exorcisms to drive out the devil and was used to fumigate houses when the plague was active.

Culpeper used it for many ailments, including snake bites, dropsy (a build-up of swelling in the tissues), coughs, cramps, gout, convulsions and to aid safe childbirth.

"The ashes of the wood are a special remedy for scurvy in the gums. The berries help the haemorrhoids or piles and kill worms in children. A lye made of the ashes of the wood, and the body bathed therewith, cures then itch, scabs and leprosy."

OTHER COMMON USES: Juniper berries are still widely used in French and southern European recipes as a complement to venison, mutton or lamb.

Juniper oil is used in the perfume industry for its masculine scent.

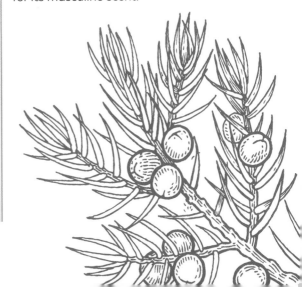

JUNIPER AND GINGER WARMING FOOT BATH

After a long autumn foraging trip along the hedgerows, there's nothing better to get the circulation back into your toes than this stimulating blend.

INGREDIENTS:

1 tsp juniper berries

1 tsp cloves

1 tbsp chopped rosehips

2 tbsp dried hibiscus

3 crushed bay leaves

Peel from ½ an orange

3 drops of ginger essential oil

Muslin bag

METHOD:

Choose a suitable bowl, just large enough for your feet. Tie all the ingredients into a muslin bag or cotton cloth and place this in the bowl, cover with boiling water, stir and leave to infuse for 10 minutes.

Add enough cold water to make it bearable to put your feet into. Soak your feet for as long as you wish.

Must not be used during pregnancy.

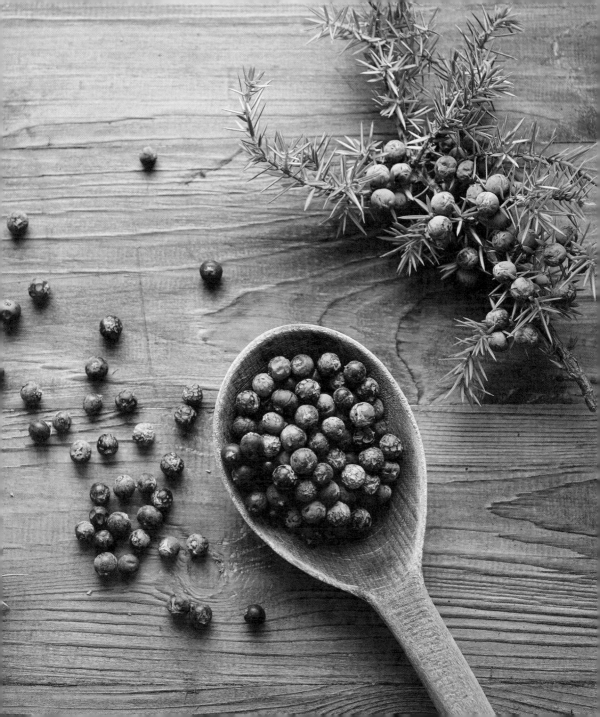

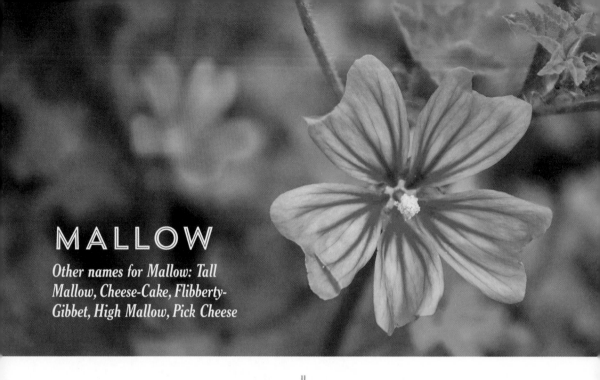

MALLOW

Other names for Mallow: Tall Mallow, Cheese-Cake, Flibberty-Gibbet, High Mallow, Pick Cheese

HOW TO IDENTIFY: These pretty mauve flowers with dark purple veins appear from June to September in sheltered, well-drained places. The ivy-shaped leaves have five to seven lobes with a covering of downy hair. The fruit are commonly called "cheeses" because they closely resemble truckles of cheese.

HISTORY: In medieval villages, it was customary for mallow flowers to be strewn in front of houses on May Day, symbolizing that marsh mallow only grows near a happy home. Marshmallow sweets were first introduced in the mid-1800s in France. They were made from the gummy sap of the mallow root, which would be sweetened, whipped and moulded into bite-sized sweets. Nowadays, marshmallows bear no trace of mallow plant, as gelatine is now the main ingredient.

FOLKLORE: The Celts, who believed in reincarnation, would protect a dead holy man by placing the cheese-shaped fruits over his eyes. This would prevent spirits from entering his body and help him to reach the afterlife safely.

In the Middle Ages, mallow was used as an antidote to aphrodisiacs and love potions. Conversely, mallow was also used to attract love.

Made into an ointment, mallow could be used to protect against demons, possession and black magic.

FOLK MEDICINE: Marsh mallow contains a soothing mucilage and so its main use was for healing sore and inflamed skin. The plant was crushed and applied to people and animals as a poultice for stings, sores, boils, insect bites, cuts and grazes.

In 1842 A. Lawson, who was a farrier, wrote:

"A neighbouring farmer had cut his thumb in a very dangerous manner and, it was got to such a pitch that his hand was swelled to twice its natural size. I recommended the use of mallows to him, gave him a little bunch out of my store, his hand was well in four days."

The plant's tiny hairs also led people to believe that it was a cure for hair loss.

OTHER COMMON USES: Marsh mallow is still used today in the treatment of coughs and sore throats, (some cough sweets still contain mallow). It is also used as a laxative, so be careful!

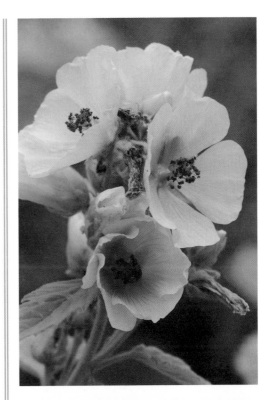

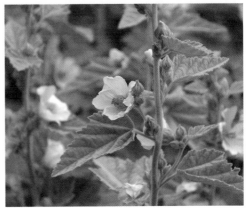

MARSH MALLOW MILK BATH

This easy recipe uses both the mallow flowers and leaves to get the utmost benefit from the soothing properties of this plant. Pick the flowers and leaves when they are at their best in the summer and dry them gently by spreading them out onto greaseproof baking paper, in an airy place, out of direct sunlight. This recipe doesn't keep, but luckily it is simple to prepare.

Makes enough for one bath.

INGREDIENTS

15 tbsp heaped chopped mallow leaves and flowers

3 tbsp organic oats

Boiling water

500 ml milk (plant-based or dairy as desired)

METHOD

Place the leaves, flowers and oats in a saucepan and cover with boiling water.

Pop a lid on the pan, turn the heat off and allow to steep for 10 minutes.

Use a potato masher to get all the gooey juices out of the mallow.

Gently heat the mixture through then add the milk and warm it through, stirring constantly.

Strain and pour into a lovely hot bath.

Use within one day.

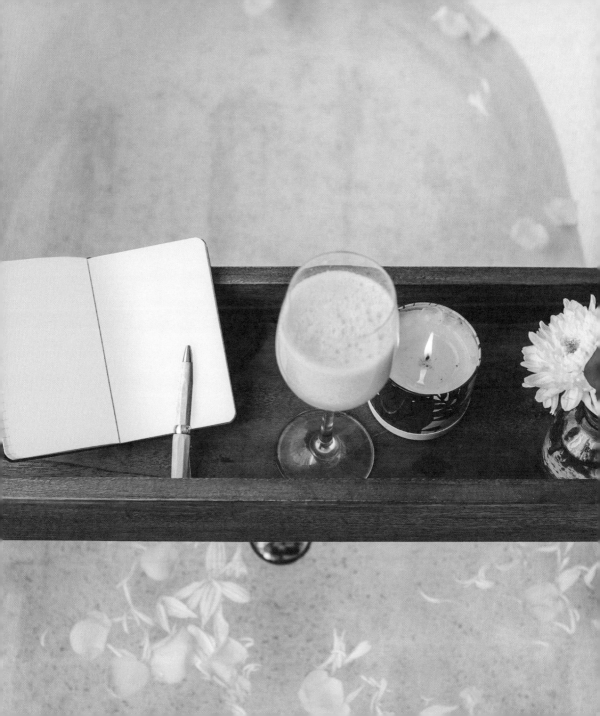

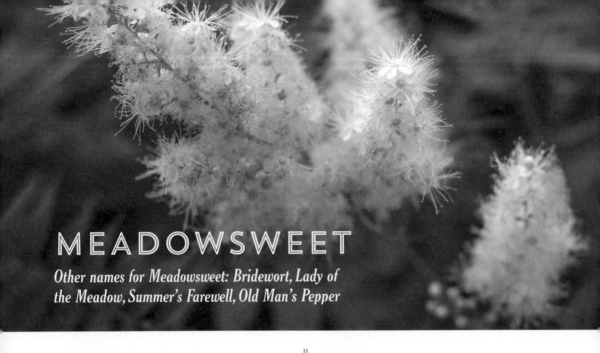

MEADOWSWEET

Other names for Meadowsweet: Bridewort, Lady of the Meadow, Summer's Farewell, Old Man's Pepper

HOW TO IDENTIFY: Meadowsweet dwells on riverbanks and in damp meadows and ditches. It flowers from June to September and is identifiable by its frothy clusters of upright, sweet-smelling, clotted cream-coloured flowers, which have an attractive vanilla/almond scent. The red stems grow to about 1.5 metres (5 feet) tall and, to my surprise, it is a member of the rose family as shown by the shape of its red tinged leaves.

HISTORY: Three of the most sacred herbs of the Druids were water mint, vervain and meadowsweet. Evidence of these has been discovered in Bronze Age burial sites in the UK, where it was found with the cremated remains of at least three people and one animal.

Considering that it doesn't generally grow in meadows, why is it called meadowsweet? Well, the answer is that during the Middle Ages, meadowsweet was a key ingredient used to flavour mead.

Meadowsweet's heady scent made it a particular favourite of Elizabeth I – she insisted that it was strewn on the floors of her bedchambers as the sweet scent would be released upon being crushed underfoot.

The seventeenth-century herbalist, Gerarde, was fond of it as a strewing herb too:

"For the smell thereof makes the heart merrie, delighting the senses, and neither does it cause headaches, or loathsome to meat, as some other sweet smelling herbs do."

FOLKLORE: A drink made from meadowsweet was considered to be a love potion and the flowers were strewn on the floor during handfastings (see May Day on page 188) to promote love and improve the overall scent of the environment. Brides' bouquets often contained meadowsweet to guarantee a happy marriage.

Should you wish to talk to faeries or acquire the gift of second sight, a good sniff of meadowsweet flowers will grant your wishes. Beware though, the heady scent was believed to induce a deep sleep from which you might not awaken or if you did, you may experience fits afterward.

FOLK MEDICINE: Along with willow, meadowsweet has been found to contain salicylic acid, the basis for aspirin. As such, it would come as no surprise to learn that it was used to make many remedies for coughs, headaches, fevers and sore throats.

Doris E. Coates wrote a fascinating book, *Tuppenny Rice and Treacle: Cottage Housekeeping 1900–1920*, which was first published in 1975, and edited with additional material by her son, Richard Coates. The book compiled recipes and housekeeping tips from the early twentieth century that had been passed down to Doris from her mother and her mother-in-law, and contained many popular recipes of the time. In her book, Doris writes that meadowsweet:

"Makes old men young and young men strong."

OTHER COMMON USES: Meadowsweet can be used to flavour wines, vinegars, beers and claret.

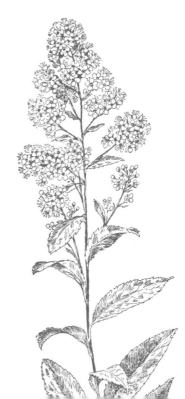

MEADOWSWEET CORDIAL

This is a lovely traditional country recipe for a floral cordial, capturing the delicious summer scent of meadowsweet in a bottle. Meadowsweet is also known for its benefits to the digestive system as well as its anti-inflammatory properties. Collect your meadowsweet on a dry day, gently shaking it to release any insects.

Makes approximately 1.5 litres.

INGREDIENTS

25 meadowsweet flower heads (the stems are bitter so leave them out)

4 unwaxed organic lemons, thinly sliced

1 kg caster sugar

1.2 litres boiling water

55 g citric acid

METHOD

Put the meadowsweet and lemons into a clean bucket or large bowl.

Dissolve the sugar in the boiling water in a large saucepan to create a syrup, then add the citric acid and stir. Carefully pour the syrup over the meadowsweet flowers and lemon, stir well, cover with a clean tea towel and leave for two to three days, stirring occasionally.

Strain the mixture through muslin and pour the liquid into sterilized bottles. Keep refrigerated or freeze in plastic bottles to be defrosted when needed.

Dilute with sparkling spring water and enjoy.

Keep refrigerated once open and use within one month.

Do not use if you are allergic to aspirin.

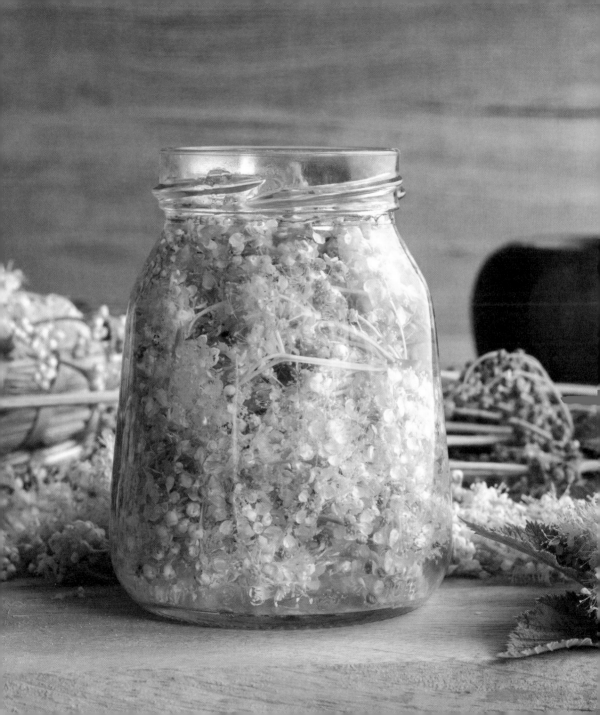

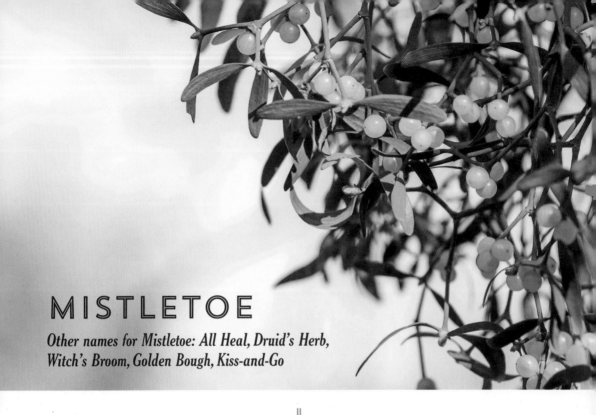

MISTLETOE

Other names for Mistletoe: All Heal, Druid's Herb, Witch's Broom, Golden Bough, Kiss-and-Go

HOW TO IDENTIFY: This parasitic plant with its globe-like form is easy to spot on the bare branches of winter trees. Mistletoe is the only plant to have distinctive forked branches, pearlescent white berries and evergreen pairs of elongated oval leaves. It most commonly grows on apple, lime and hawthorn trees.

All parts are poisonous to animals and it is not recommended for human consumption unless prescribed by a medical herbalist. Wear gloves to avoid contact.

HISTORY: It was thought that mistletoe grew from bird droppings: *"mistel"* means dung in Anglo Saxon, so mistletoe is said to translate as "dung on a twig".

Mistletoe was considered sacred by the Druids and other pagan religions, especially if it was growing on their hallowed oak trees. The most powerful magic wands used by the Druids were made from oak trees that had mistletoe growing on them.

The Druids cut mistletoe using a golden sickle on the sixth night of the new moon after the winter solstice. It was not allowed to touch the ground as it would lose its magical powers, hence it would be caught in a cloak. The chief Druid would then divide the branches into many sprigs and distribute them for hanging over doorways to protect against thunder, lightning and other evils. Due to the pagan association with mistletoe, it was banned from being used as Christmas decorations in churches.

FOLKLORE: In some countries, sprigs were placed in the stable to keep livestock safe from local witches. In England and Wales, farmers hung a bunch of mistletoe in the byre of the first cow that calved to ensure the health and milk production of the herd for the year.

Kissing under the mistletoe used to be interpreted as a promise to marry. Every time a girl is kissed under the mistletoe a berry should be picked, this ensures that she will marry and have a child within the coming year. If kissing under the mistletoe wasn't successful, it was sometimes worn around the arm or neck to ensure fertility.

All the mistletoe used to decorate the house must be burned before Twelfth Night, otherwise couples will quarrel and definitely not marry.

FOLK MEDICINE: During medieval times, mistletoe was known to rural people as the best cure for barren women and, in Somerset, it was used to create a vile tasting tea to cure measles. Mistletoe can only be used under the supervision of a medical herbalist.

Many illnesses were thought to be caused by the forces of evil. Mistletoe's status as a sacred plant meant that it was regarded as a panacea to cure all ailments.

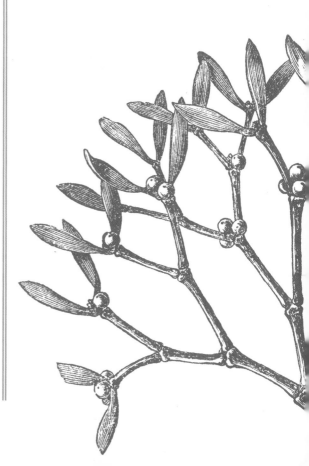

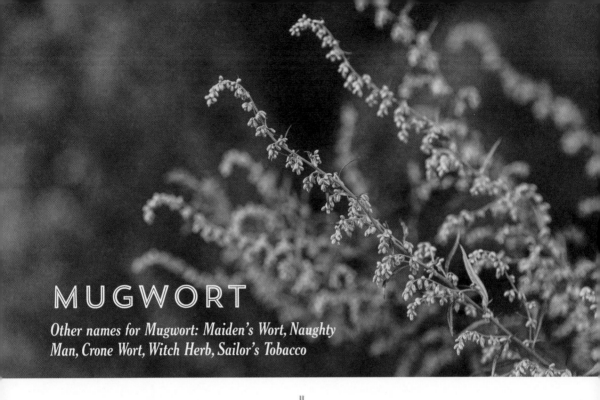

MUGWORT

Other names for Mugwort: Maiden's Wort, Naughty Man, Crone Wort, Witch Herb, Sailor's Tobacco

HOW TO IDENTIFY: This hardy plant grows on wasteland and verges and it can grow up to 2 metres (6½ feet) tall. The leaves are delicate and finely lobed, dark green on the uppermost side and covered in dense silvery hairs on the underside. Mugwort is in bloom from June to September, with tiny clusters of whitish-green flowers and a distinct fragrance of sage.

HISTORY: Dried mugwort was burned during rituals and ceremonies and was one of the nine sacred herbs of the Anglo Saxons. Medieval ale called *"gruit"* was brewed using mugwort, myrtle and yarrow, and was to be served in large *"mugs"*; it is thought this is how the plant got its name. However, other theories suggest that the name comes from the plant's ability to deter midges and moths or *"muggia"*.

Thirteenth-century Welsh doctors, known in folklore as the Physicians of Myddfai, knew the usefulness of mugwort as an insecticide:

> *"to destroy flies, let the mugwort be put in a place where they are frequent and they will die."*

FOLKLORE: St John the Baptist is believed to have worn a girdle of mugwort around his waist to protect himself from the devil when he went into the wilderness. In medieval times, it was thought that if you dug under a mugwort plant on Midsummer's Eve you would find a "coal", carrying this with you guaranteed protection from witchcraft, lightning, plague, infected swellings and burning.

Bunches of mugwort were hung above doorways to protect against evil entering the home. As recently as the nineteenth century, German people wore headdresses of mugwort and vervain while looking at a bonfire through bunches of larkspur to keep their eyes healthy for another year. As they left the fireside, they threw their headdresses into the fire saying:

"May all my ill luck depart and be burnt up with these."

Mugwort was often used to predict the future, with an infusion being used to clean crystal balls and scrying mirrors. Burning incense made from mugwort and sandalwood was also used to aid concentration for the psychic.

FOLK MEDICINE: Known as *"mater herbarum"*, mother of herbs, mugwort was traditionally used for childbirth, fertility and virginity.

Culpeper wrote:

"This is an herb of Venus. Its tops, leaves and flowers are full of virtue, they are aromatic, and most safe and excellent in female disorders."

Mugwort was widely used for "women's problems", for balancing the monthly cycle and helping with cases of difficult childbirth.

Thirteenth-century Roman soldiers wrapped mugwort around their feet to prevent weariness while marching.

In 1656, the celebrated botanist William Coles wrote:

"And if a footman take mugwort and put it into his shoes in the morning, he may goe forty miles before noon and not be weary."

OTHER COMMON USES: Tea made with mugwort can be used as an environmentally friendly plant spray to repel insects. Care is needed as it can also inhibit growth. Dried mugwort can be hung in a wardrobe to deter moths.

PEACEFUL SLEEP PILLOW

Dream pillows can be personalized to create a herbal mix that is perfect
for individual sleep problems. These make lovely gifts for friends and family
and can be made using scraps of cotton cloth or ready-made pouches.

INGREDIENTS

Natural fabric or
small organza pouch

Herbs of choice

Needle and thread

METHOD

Make your pillow by folding your fabric in half and sewing up
two of the three open sides. Fill the bag loosely with your chosen
herbal mix and sew the remaining edge shut.

Place under your pillow and enjoy the pleasant herbal aromas as
you sleep.

Herb suggestions:

- **Mugwort:** Good for people who want to remember their dreams, can make your dreams colourful and protect you from nightmares.
- **Chamomile:** For calm, peaceful sleep. Good for insomnia and can ease anxiety and fears.
- **Lemon balm:** Calming and uplifting, and can also help with stress, depression and anxiety.
- **Lavender:** Just a small amount added to your dream pillow can ease headaches and aid relaxation.
- **Rosemary:** Helps you to remember dreams and recollect things that have been lost or forgotten.
- **Rose:** Brings a feeling of love and warmth to your dreams.
- **Hops:** For deep sleep and relaxation.

Not recommended during pregnancy.

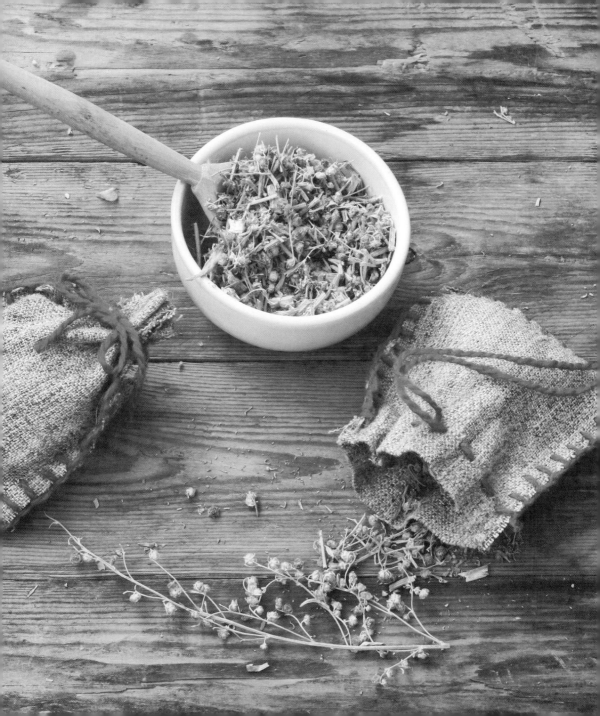

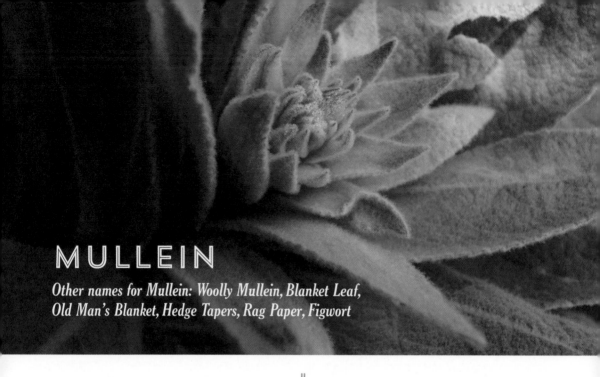

MULLEIN

Other names for Mullein: Woolly Mullein, Blanket Leaf,
Old Man's Blanket, Hedge Tapers, Rag Paper, Figwort

HOW TO IDENTIFY: The distinctive flower spikes of the mullein grow to over 2 metres (6½ feet) tall and can be found on railway embankments, open fields or anywhere that is dry and sunny. The silvery leaves have soft hairs with the feel of thick felt – no surprise then that they have often been used as nature's toilet paper for people caught short in the countryside! Pale yellow, saucer-shaped flowers climb around the flower spike and are in bloom throughout summer.

HISTORY: The dried-out leaves and stems were used by the Romans as tinder to light fires and the folded leaves replaced wicks in oil lamps. In medieval times, whole dried plants were carried to light a funeral procession. The sedative properties of the seeds were used to the advantage of poachers who sprinkled them onto rivers to intoxicate fish, making them easier to catch.

The medieval poor would line their shoes with the soft leaves in winter for extra warmth, and they also served as a natural infant's nappy. Despite their softness, the fine hairs on the mullein leaves can cause irritation. Sometimes known as "Quaker rouge", young girls would use the leaves to redden their cheeks.

Many flowers soaked in water produced a hair dye for Roman ladies to turn their hair yellow, and soap made from the ashes of mullein was used to colour grey hairs.

FOLKLORE: Witches were purported to take to the skies on mullein spikes to reach their night time coven meetings. These gatherings would be illuminated by mullein candles and lanterns.

As with many hedgerow plants, mullein was used to test the faithfulness of a lover: the plant was bent over to point at the lover's house, if it straightened up again, then all was well, however if it died, their love was untrue.

FOLK MEDICINE: Leaves and flowers were combined with other herbs and made into a tea to ease coughs and colds – the fine hairs were removed as they caused irritation. Leaves placed in shoes were supposed to ward off infections and ease aching feet, as well as keeping the feet warm.

OTHER COMMON USES: To remove splinters and draw out boils, lay a mullein leaf in a dish, pour over a little boiling water and leave to cool. Wrap around the affected part and secure with a bandage.

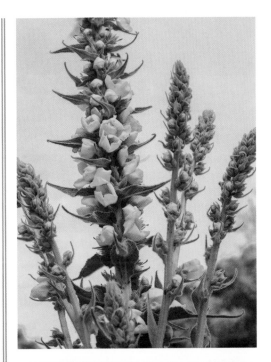

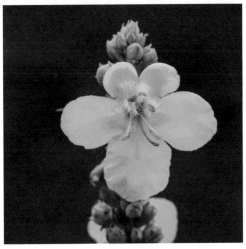

MULLEIN AND GARLIC EAR DROPS

This is a useful first aid remedy for ear ache, as mullein has soothing properties and garlic is a natural antibiotic. Do not use if you suspect that your eardrum is perforated, instead seek medical help. Not recommended for prolonged use.

INGREDIENTS

2 tbsp washed mullein flowers

2 tbsp organic garlic, minced

Organic olive oil

Muslin

Jar

Small glass dropper bottle

METHOD

Place mullein and garlic in a heatproof bowl and add just enough olive oil to cover. Put some water in the bottom of a small pan, place the bowl containing the olive oil mixture on top and warm gently on the cooker to infuse for 20–30 minutes.

Strain through muslin to remove all solids.

Transfer into a sterilized jar. Keep your oil in the fridge to preserve freshness.

Rub a little of the oil onto the inside of your wrist to check that you are not allergic to any of the ingredients.

To use: Pour into the sterilized dropper bottle and warm up the oil by rubbing it between your hands. Pop three to four drops into the affected ear as needed. Use within one month.

Do not use during pregnancy.

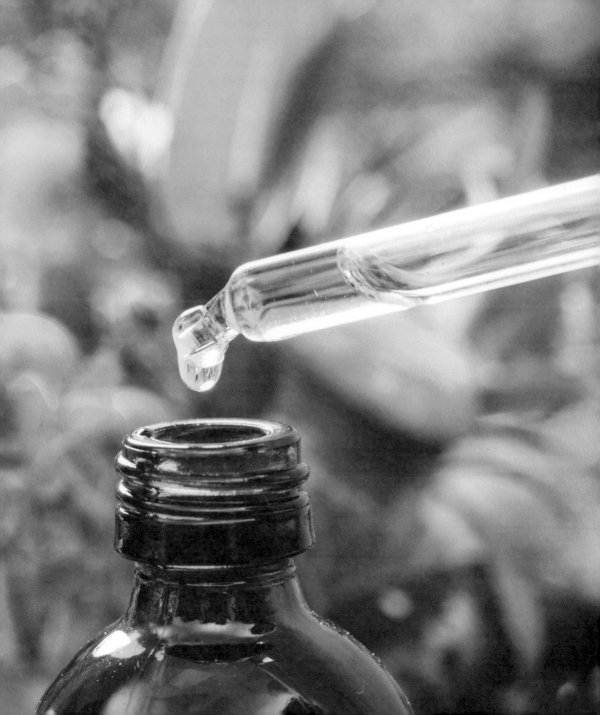

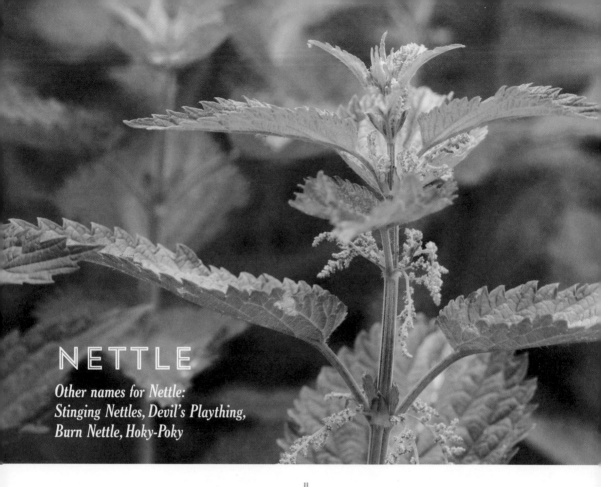

NETTLE

Other names for Nettle:
Stinging Nettles, Devil's Plaything,
Burn Nettle, Hoky-Poky

HOW TO IDENTIFY: Growing everywhere it would seem where there might be vulnerable bare arms and legs, nettles are often felt before they are seen! Dark green, hairy, heart-shaped stingy leaves are arranged set opposite each other in pairs along a tall, straight stem. The flowers form at the base of the leaves and are greenish-white with yellow anthers.

HISTORY: The nettle plant contains strong fibres that have been spun since the Bronze Age for making cloth and cord.

During World War I, when cotton was scarce, nettle fibre was cultivated on a huge scale to be made into uniforms for German and Austrian soldiers. Green dye made from the nettles helped to make camouflage uniforms for the British army during World

War II, and there were even plans to construct aircraft wings from nettle fibres. During rationing, many people used nettles in their cooking as they were a good source of vitamin C and iron.

FOLKLORE: Nettles were used to thrash the devil out of poor souls believed to be possessed. Holding a nettle during a thunderstorm – if you can bear the stings – will prevent you from getting struck by lightning. Carry yarrow with it and it will help you become fearless – very useful during a thunderstorm!

To stimulate hair growth, try combing nettle juice into your hair; this will make hair soft and glossy, and prevent it from falling out.

FOLK MEDICINE: It was believed that a fever could be cured by picking a nettle up by its roots while reciting the name of the sick person and also the names of their parents. An old remedy for rheumatism and arthritis involved whipping the affected joints with fresh nettles – this has been proven to give some pain relief, despite a nasty nettle rash!

In the seventeenth century, earache was soothed by dripping nettle juice into ears. Mix nettle juice with egg white and rub onto temples to cure insomnia or use it to ease burns and rashes.

OTHER COMMON USES: Full of vitamins, protein and iron, nettles make a useful substitute for spinach – don't worry, the stings completely disappear after cooking.

Today, the chlorophyll of nettle is used as a green dye and is known as the food colourant E140.

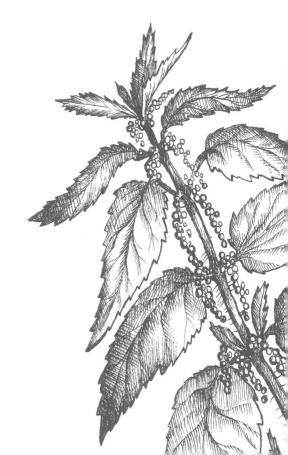

NETTLE HAIR TONIC

Use as a final rinse to stimulate hair growth and strengthen the hair. Remember to wear long sleeves and gloves to gather your nettles and forage away from popular dog-walking areas.

Makes enough for two applications on short hair or one application for longer hair.

INGREDIENTS

1 large bunch of fresh nettle tops

500 ml water

500 ml white wine (or apple cider) vinegar

1 tbsp of aromatic fresh or dried herbs of your choice (chamomile or sunflower petals for fair hair, sage or rosemary for dark hair, calendula or marigold for red hair)

METHOD

Put the nettles in a large pan with the water and vinegar and bring to a simmer for 2 hours.

Stir in the herbs; essential oils could be added too.

Allow the liquid to cool.

Strain through muslin and bottle.

Use within one week.

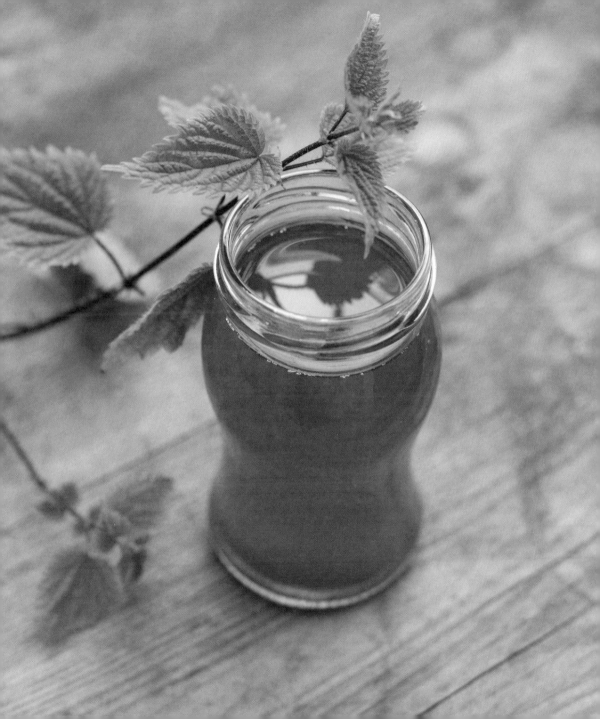

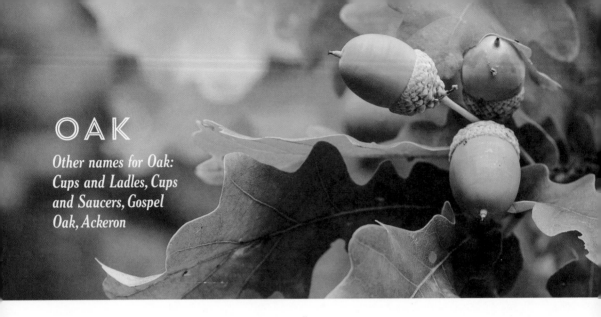

OAK

*Other names for Oak:
Cups and Ladles, Cups
and Saucers, Gospel
Oak, Ackeron*

HOW TO IDENTIFY: This well-loved deciduous tree can grow to well over 30 metres (about 100 feet) tall. It has a broad-spreading crown that allows light to fall on the woodland floor below.

The lobed leaves burst into life in bunches around May, followed by long yellow catkins that blow in the breeze, distributing their pollen. Acorn fruits follow the catkins, which ripen to a nutty brown and fall to the ground in the autumn when they are gathered by hungry squirrels and other hedgerow dwellers.

HISTORY: The oak is such an important tree in shaping Britain's history. Prized for its strength and durability it was, and still is, used in the construction of houses, churches and ships. Until the middle of the nineteenth century, all ships for the Royal Navy were constructed from oak, giving rise to the tree's nickname of "the wooden walls of old England".

Historically, oak has been used to make barrels to store wine and spirits in, and the bark was an essential ingredient in the leather tanning industry.

Gospel oaks were planted to mark parish borders, the custom of "beating the bounds" is still carried out on Ascension Day, the fortieth day of Easter. Parishioners walk the boundaries of the parish, possibly beating them with willow sticks, to remind everyone of their location and ensure that a neighbouring parish hasn't acquired some of their land.

FOLKLORE: Be warned: never cut down an oak tree, you will hear it screaming and be dead yourself within a year! If you must cut down an oak, however, you can protect yourself by carrying a bible in your pocket and singing psalms as you work.

Ancient trees were regarded as having great powers and dreaming of oak trees foretells of a long and wealthy life. Float two acorn cups on water to predict if your love affair will be long lasting. If the acorn cups drift together, you will be married, if they float apart...

Cords of window blinds were customarily carved into the shape of acorns to prevent lightning from entering through the window, as it was believed that oak trees never got struck by lightning. A protective amulet made by binding two equal-sized pieces of oak together with red cord to form a cross was suspended in the house to protect the occupants from evil.

Hollow oaks, known as "bull oaks" were said to house faeries, spirits and demons, and people passing by were warned to turn their coats inside out in an attempt to avoid being bewitched by faery magic in this traditional rhyme:

"Turn your cloaks, for fairy folks are in old oaks."

FOLK MEDICINE: The oak played a significant role in symbolic healing, especially in cases of fever. The patient was taken to a crossroads where an oak was growing, the illness could then be "transferred" into the oak tree. A lock of the patient's hair was nailed to the trunk and pulled out with a swift jerk transferring the fever and the hair into the tree.

Grated acorn in white wine is said to relieve "the stitch" and a decoction of the bark was used as a gargle to treat diarrhoea and as a wash for piles.

Culpeper writes:

"The water that is found in hollow places of old oaks is very effectual against any foul smelling scabs."

Catching a falling oak leaf in the autumn will prevent you from catching a cold, and oak logs burned in a sick person's room will draw out all their ailments. Carrying an acorn in your pocket or handbag will prevent ageing as well as increasing your virility.

OTHER COMMON USES: Surprisingly, many things can be made from acorns, from coffee substitutes to acorn flour. They can also be useful in art and craft projects.

ACORN CUP FLOATING FAERY CANDLES

This is a delightfully time-consuming craft that involves foraging for lovely large acorn cups, but don't use cracked or chipped ones as the wax will leak out. I'm lucky enough to have a friendly beekeeper in my village who gives me his unwanted beeswax for this craft – if you ask around you might be able to find one too.

INGREDIENTS

As many acorn cups as you can gather

Beeswax (or any other candle wax)

Candle wicks

Dried herbs and flowers

METHOD

Using a hot glue gun, secure a wick into the bottom of each acorn cup.

Using a double boiler with water in the bottom, carefully melt the beeswax.

Pour melted wax to the top of the acorn cup using a teaspoon, but be careful, it's hot!

It will set fairly quickly but you can push it into an old piece of polystyrene to keep it upright as it cools. Snip off any excess wick that pokes out over the top.

Float in water in a wide, flat bowl scattered with dried herbs, and light carefully.

Keep the candles in the fridge before using as this makes them burn a little slower.

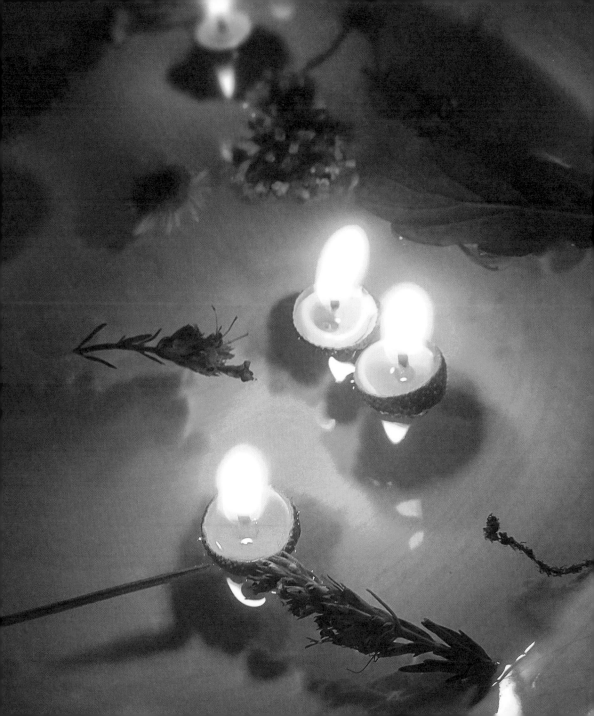

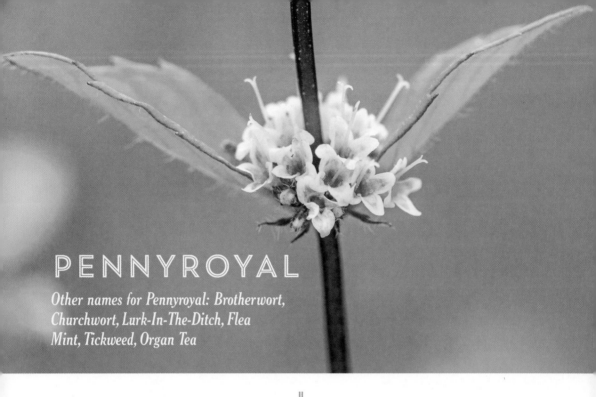

PENNYROYAL

Other names for Pennyroyal: Brotherwort, Churchwort, Lurk-In-The-Ditch, Flea Mint, Tickweed, Organ Tea

HOW TO IDENTIFY: The pennyroyal is the most diminutive of the mint family. It hugs the ground and can be found invading poorly drained soil on the sides of ditches and marshlands. It gives off a lovely peppermint aroma when trodden on, making it quite easy to find by smell rather than sight. Pretty lavender blue flowers appear in whorls in the summer, with leaves that are jagged and grow opposite one another.

HISTORY: Pennyroyal was often used as a strewing herb and infused to mop floors as it was known to have insect repellent properties. It is written in *The Compleat Herbal of Physical Plants* by John Pechey of the College of Physicians in London, published in 1694, that:

> *"The fresh herb wrap'd in cloth and laid in a bed, drives away fleas; but it must be renewed once a week."*

Sailors in the sixteenth century used pennyroyal to sweeten and purify their drinking water while at sea. Mixed with wormwood, pennyroyal was a cure for seasickness and when sprinkled onto the ocean, it was believed to calm the seas.

In Yorkshire it was called "pudding-yerb" as it was picked to flavour black puddings and as an ingredient for stuffing.

FOLKLORE: Drowned bees could be revived by placing them on a bed of pennyroyal ashes and putting the herb inside the hive discouraged the bees from swarming.

Wearing pennyroyal not only gave you protection from the evil eye – very important in medieval times – but also stopped anyone from arguing with you. Keep a bowl of pennyroyal somewhere in the house to stop family quarrels. Travellers on long journeys placed pennyroyal into their shoes to combat tiredness.

Pennyroyal is known to be a magical herb. It was burned by witches to help them explore the border between life and death, and also used in the embalming process to aid transition to the spirit world.

FOLK MEDICINE: Pennyroyal water was made from the leaves and prescribed for a variety of ailments including nervous conditions, hysterical complaints, chills and to promote the sweating out of colds and fevers, as noted by John Gerarde, sixteenth-century botanist and herbalist:

"A garland of pennyroyal made and worn about the head is of great force against the swimming of the head and the pains and giddiness thereof."

Pennyroyal was often used to bring on menstruation and ease monthly cramps; this led to it also being taken to bring on miscarriages for unwanted pregnancies.

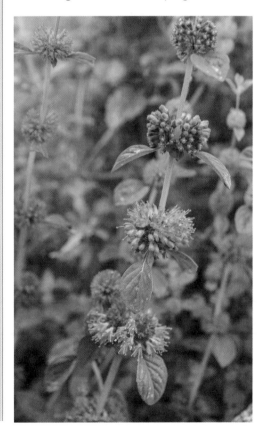

MOTH REPELLENT WARDROBE SACHETS

Clothing moths are not attracted to light, preferring to burrow themselves away where they won't be disturbed. Hanging these sachets among the clothes in your wardrobe will deter them from making a home in your best woollen jumper. All the ingredients are known for their insect repellent properties and are readily available online.

INGREDIENTS

50 g dried pennyroyal*

50 g dried lavender

50 g dried tansy

50 g dried mint

10 whole cloves

10 black peppercorns

1 tbsp dried thyme

1 tbsp dried rosemary

2 drops lemon essential oil

Drawstring cotton or organza bag

METHOD

Mix all the herbs together then add the lemon oil and mix again.

Fill your drawstring bag and hang it in your wardrobe.

Store any unused mixture in an airtight container for future use.

*Pennyroyal is not to be used during pregnancy.

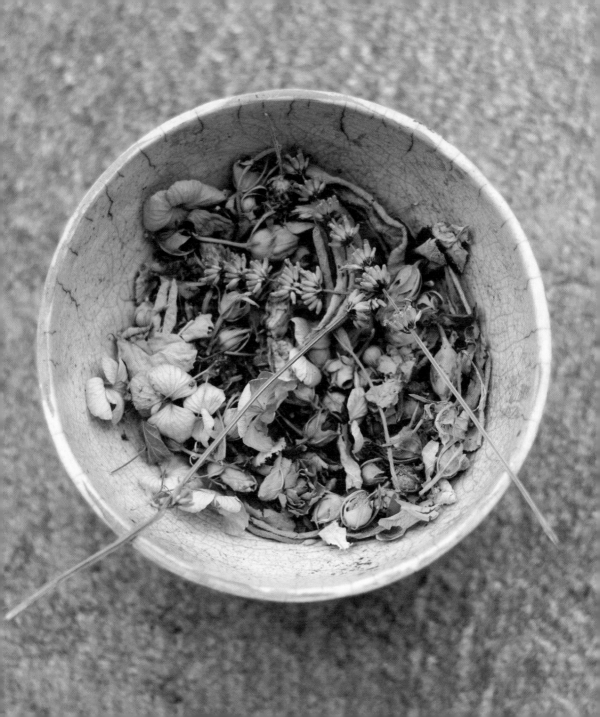

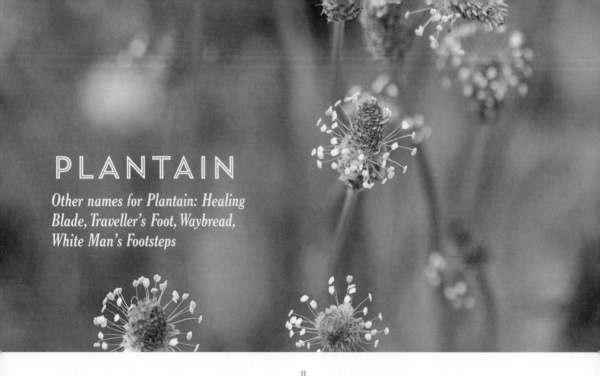

PLANTAIN

Other names for Plantain: Healing Blade, Traveller's Foot, Waybread, White Man's Footsteps

HOW TO IDENTIFY: A ubiquitous perennial plant found in lawns, at roadsides and on footpaths. Described by some as a short, fat, ugly weed, the plantain is actually one of the best healing herbs on Earth.

The broad, oval-shaped leaves grow in a rosette with distinctive stringy veins running from the bottom to the top.

The long, slender flower stalks grow from the central core with many tiny greenish-yellow flowers that produce hundreds of seeds.

HISTORY: The plantain is often found growing on paths and, as such, it is trodden on frequently. The tough leaves lie flat and allow it to survive the heaviest of tramplings. This led to the Native Americans using the name "White Man's Footsteps" – the seeds were picked up and brought over on the soles of the shoes of the White settlers and proceeded to spread everywhere the White men travelled.

FOLKLORE: A necklace made from the plantain will shield you from being abducted by faeries and an amulet will protect you from insect stings and snake bites.

In the seventeenth century, John Aubrey wrote:

"The last summer, on the day of St John the Baptist... I saw there about two or three and twenty young women, most of them well habited, on their knees very busy, as if they had been weeding. I could not presently learn what the matter was; at last a young man told me, that they were looking for the coal under the root of a plantain, to put under their head that night, and they should dream of who would be their husbands."

FOLK MEDICINE: Our Anglo Saxon ancestors prepared a "Nine Herbs Charm" invoking Woden, the chief god of the Anglo Saxons; this gave the healer reciting the incantation the ability to cure the sick. Plantain was included in the charm as well as mugwort, lamb's cress, betony, chamomile, nettle, crab apple, chervil and fennel. The herbs were pounded and made into a paste with ashes and egg and applied to the wound while chanting the charm. Worn in the shoes, the mixture eased the weariness of long-distance walkers and tied around the head with red cord, it cured headaches.

Historically, it has mostly been used for its ability to treat infection, cuts, stings, bites, varicose ulcers, sore eyes and ears and even broken bones.

In Shakespeare's *Love's Labour's Lost*, Costard calls for:

"O, sir, plantain, a plain plantain! ... no salve, sir, but a plantain!"

to mend his broken shin.

OTHER COMMON USES: Young leaves can be put in salads, although they can be rather bitter. Still valuable as a traditional remedy for insect or nettle stings, the leaves are antibacterial and anti-inflammatory. Chew the leaves before using on the skin as the enzymes in saliva help to release the active constituents needed for healing.

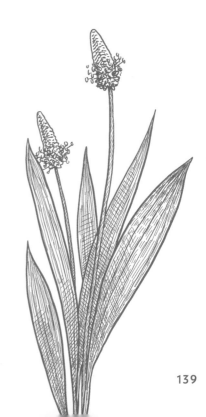

PLANTAIN FIRST AID OINTMENT

The healing properties of this plant make it the perfect remedy to have on hand when out and about. Use for nettle stings, mosquito bites, bee and wasp stings, sunburn, eczema and suchlike. Plantain leaves contain some water, which could cause your ointment to go rancid. To limit this risk, use only leaves picked on a dry day and make sure that your jar is completely moisture-free too.

Makes approximately 1 full jam jar.

INGREDIENTS

A good handful of plantain leaves from an area that is pesticide free

250 ml olive oil

25 g natural beeswax

10 drops of lavender oil (optional)

METHOD

Clean your leaves with a paper towel and discard any that are brown or blemished. Roughly chop up the leaves in a food processor, add the oil and whizz again briefly.

Pour the oil into a large heatproof jam jar. Place the jam jar in a saucepan and fill the pan with enough water so that it comes about halfway up the outside of the jar. Set the heat to maintain a low simmer for 2 hours to infuse. Don't let all the water boil away!

Strain out the plantain leaves – the oil will be a pale shade of green. Return to the jar, add the beeswax and melt it by putting it back into the pan of warm water.

Stir in the lavender oil if using and pour into clean, dry containers. Allow to cool before popping the lid on.

Use within six months.

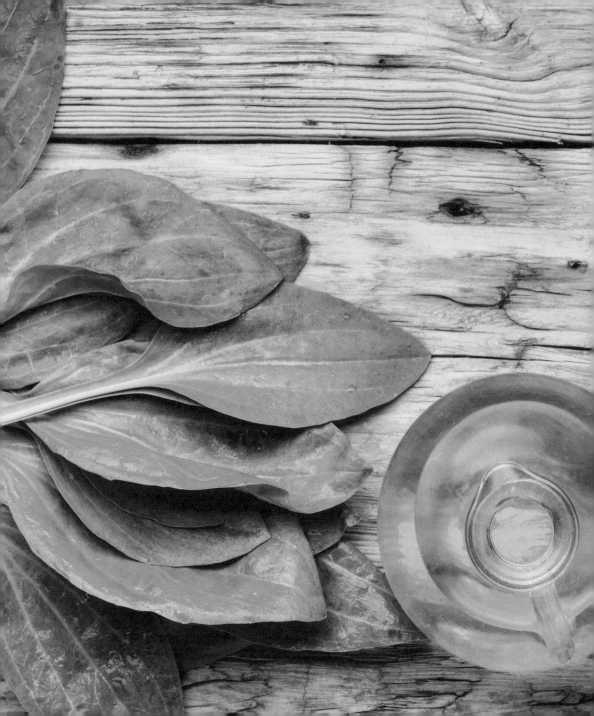

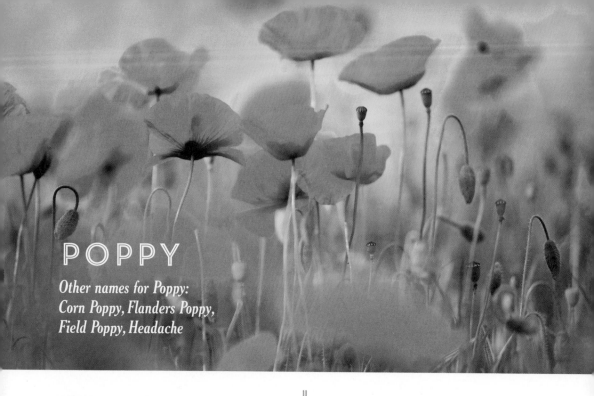

POPPY

Other names for Poppy:
Corn Poppy, Flanders Poppy,
Field Poppy, Headache

HOW TO IDENTIFY: The wild poppy grows in disturbed soil. The papery thin scarlet flower barely lasts a day on its tall hairy stem.

HISTORY: The red corn poppy has become a very powerful symbol of Remembrance Day. The ground was churned up on the battlefields of France and so poppies bloomed in abundance. The flowers also proliferated on the graves of the fallen.

Inspired by the death of a friend, Canadian physician and Lieutenant-Colonel John McCrae wrote his powerfully poignant poem, "In Flanders Fields", during World War I:

> *"In Flanders Fields the poppies blow,*
> *Between the crosses, row on row,*
> *That mark our place; and in the sky,*
> *The larks still bravely singing, fly.*
> *Scarce heard amid the guns below,*
> *We are the dead. Short days ago*
> *We lived, felt dawn, saw sunset glow,*
> *Loved and were loved, and now we lie*
> *In Flanders Fields."*

FOLKLORE: It seems that the poppy has always been associated with warnings of injury or harm. Pick or smell a poppy flower and you could quite possibly be struck by lightning, become blind or, rather worryingly, wake up covered in warts. Maybe this particular superstition was concocted to stop children from trampling all over precious cornfields where poppies once flourished.

Despite the poppy's bleak historical associations, poppy petals could also be used in the popular pastime of love divination: place a poppy petal in your left palm, strike it with your right palm. If there is no sound, unfortunately there is no love either.

To dream of your future husband, scatter poppy seeds behind you on St Andrews Day. For fertility, wear a necklace of poppy seed heads – be careful though, poppy seeds put in a new bride's shoes will render her infertile.

If you are being chased by a demon, poppy seeds thrown in its path will distract it long enough for you to escape because demons feel compelled to count things. The seeds are also good for keeping vampires away.

FOLK MEDICINE: The petals and seeds are known to have mild sedative properties and were used to good effect by both land girls and tired mothers during World War II.

OTHER COMMON USES: Red poppy petals can be used to brighten up your salad, and the seeds are delicious baked into cakes and bread.

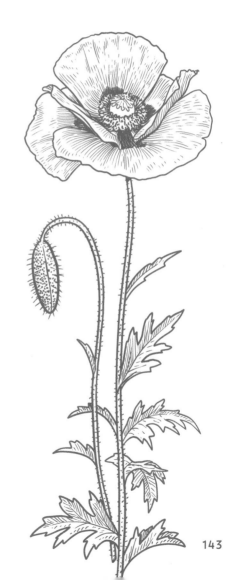

POPPY SEED FACIAL SCRUB

Essential fatty acids and antioxidants in poppy seeds will help to give skin a natural glow. Lemon juice is antibacterial and can reduce redness and brighten the complexion.

Makes approximately 180 g.

INGREDIENTS

100 g caster sugar

30 g poppy seeds

Finely grated zest from 1 unwaxed lemon

50 g coconut oil

2 tsp lemon juice

METHOD

Mix the poppy seeds, sugar and lemon zest together.

Gently melt the coconut oil and pour into the sugar mixture, add the lemon juice and combine.

The mixture should resemble wet sand.

Rub a small amount between the palms and gently apply to wet skin using a circular motion.

Rinse and pat dry.

Use within one month.

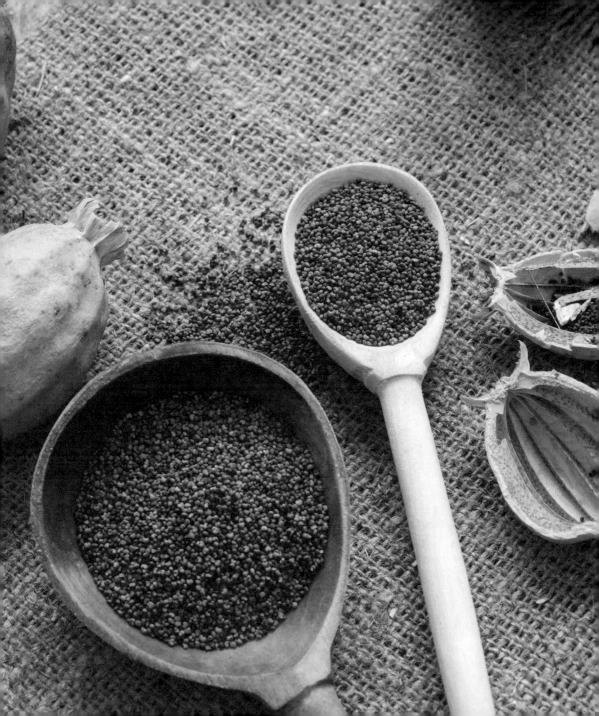

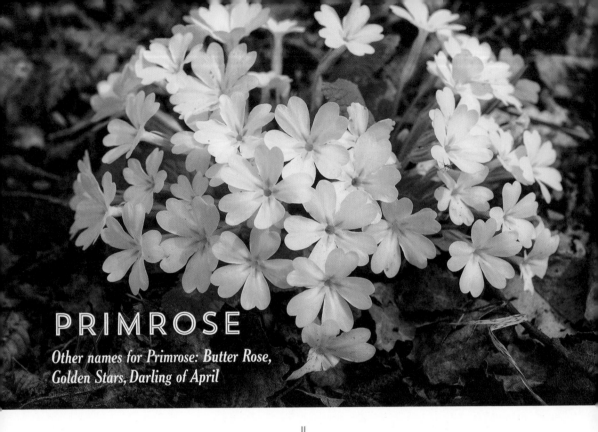

PRIMROSE

Other names for Primrose: Butter Rose,
Golden Stars, Darling of April

HOW TO IDENTIFY: This pretty woodland perennial heralds the start of spring. It grows in neat clumps with pale lemon flowers dotted with a deeper yellow or orange centre. The single flowers have five notched petals on upright furry stalks. The crinkly, wrinkly, short-stemmed leaves have hairy undersides that form a rosette at the base of the plant.

HISTORY: Primroses were so popular in Victorian times that country people would gather them into posies and send them to London to sell to city dwellers. Unfortunately, this could be why we just don't see so many primroses in the wild nowadays.

FOLKLORE: Some folklore credits primroses with the ability to let people see faeries, either by eating their petals or by placing a bunch on a faery rock or faery mound. In Ireland, the flowers were scattered by the byre to stop faeries from stealing the milk. In many counties it is considered unlucky to bring primrose flowers into the house and a primrose flowering in the winter was taken as an omen of death.

Bunches of primroses were hung in cowsheds during the Celtic festival of Beltane to protect the cattle from witches. Churches were decorated with primroses and they would also be placed on doorsteps to prevent witches and bad faeries from entering.

On the contrary, some folklore says that bringing primroses into the house can be a good thing. The primrose has long been associated with the hatching of eggs, both goose and hen. If a bunch of primroses was gathered, the corresponding number of eggs would hatch. A broody hen's clutch would traditionally number thirteen so you should gather a minimum of thirteen primroses.

Parents would sew primroses into the pillows of their children to ensure eternal love and loyalty. When worn, primroses were also believed to cure madness and to attract love.

FOLK MEDICINE: Healing salves for skin conditions and burns were traditionally made from primrose flowers. The leaves were infused into boiled water to make soothing eyewash or a gargle for sore throats. Juice from primroses and cowslips was applied to soften wrinkles, their crinkly leaves resembled wrinkly skin so it was a reasonable assumption that it would work.

When boiled with lard, primroses were made into a salve for cuts and minor wounds. Primrose tea is purported to alleviate anxiety, and the roots and plant were made into cough medicine.

OTHER COMMON USES: The flowers can be used to make a country wine but are also crystallized (see page 172) for use as cake decorations.

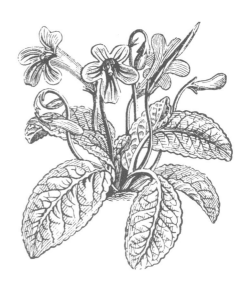

PRIMROSE MERINGUES

Pick primroses or primulas from your garden to make these unusual sweet treats and leave the wild ones for everyone to enjoy.

Makes approximately 8 meringues.

INGREDIENTS

4 large egg whites

240 g caster sugar

10 fresh primrose flowers, chopped

METHOD

Preheat the oven to 150°C (300°F).

Whisk the egg whites with 60 g of the sugar until it forms soft peaks.

Still whisking, gradually add the rest of the sugar, keeping the soft peaks.

Gently fold in the chopped primrose flowers.

Line a baking sheet with baking paper.

Spoon or pipe the meringue mixture to form eight mounds, making sure that they have space to spread.

Bake for 45 minutes until firm to the touch and the palest golden brown.

Leave to cool, then carefully peel away from the paper.

Sandwich together with whipped cream or lemon curd.

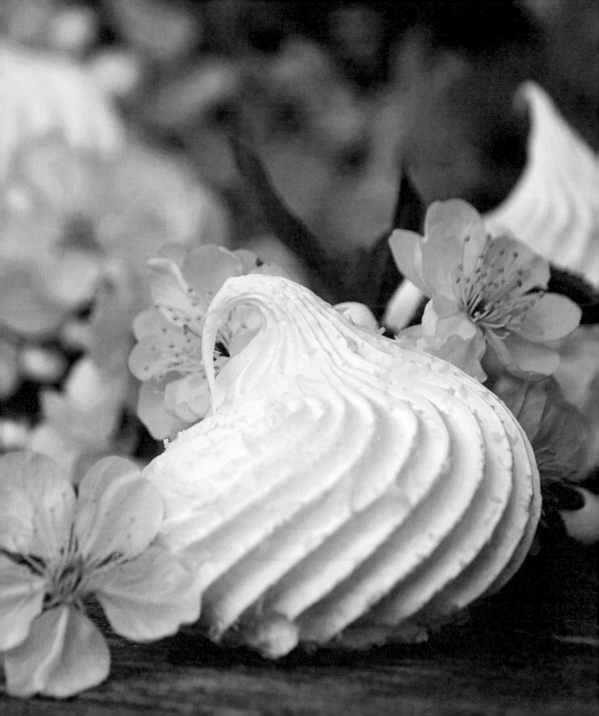

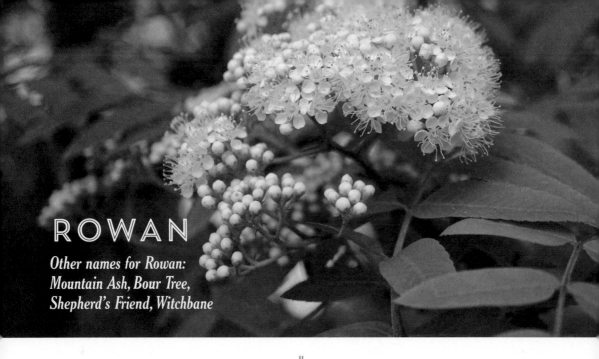

ROWAN

Other names for Rowan:
Mountain Ash, Bour Tree,
Shepherd's Friend, Witchbane

HOW TO IDENTIFY: The rowan is a small, grey-barked tree that is common in rocky places and dry, wooded areas. The leaves are feather-like, comprising of five to eight pairs of distinctive, serrated leaflets.

The flower heads, which appear from May to June, are buttery white with five petals on flat branched clusters. In autumn, the leaves turn a brilliant flame colour, dangling with round, fleshy, scarlet fruits.

HISTORY: Rowan wood is hard-wearing and tough, making it a good choice for tool handles, walking sticks, spinning wheels and spindles.

Druids dyed their ceremonial garments black using the bark and berries, and the twigs were also used to make wands, runes and divining rods.

Traditionally, the berries have been used to make a variety of alcoholic drinks. The Scots brewed wine and spirits, the Welsh preferred to brew ale, the Irish mead, and the English cider.

FOLKLORE: Rowan Tree Witch Day was held on the Celtic festival of Beltane. Branches were cut from the tree in the belief that they would give protection from witches for the coming year. Rowan branches were placed over beds to ensure restful sleep, near wells to protect the water and into milk churns to stop milk from being stolen. Crosses were made and tied with red thread to be stitched into clothing for protection.

As Christianity spread, wood for protective amulets was gathered on Good Friday while reciting this spell from *Plant Lore, Legends, and Lyrics: Embracing the Myths, Traditions, Superstitions, and Folk-Lore of the Plant Kingdom*, written in 1884 by Richard Folkard:

"From Witches and Wizards,
and long-tailed Buzzards,
And things that run in the hedge-bottoms,
Good Lord, deliver us!"

On May Day, farmers drove their sheep and lambs through rowan hoops and made yokes for their oxen to avoid bewitching.

Druids believed that wine made from rowan berries would grant them the gift of second sight.

FOLK MEDICINE: Rowan berries and apples were cooked and passed through a sieve to make a gargle for whooping cough.

The leaves could be carried or made into a tea for rheumatism or burned and inhaled for asthma. The tea was also used to ease the pains of childbirth and help to expel the afterbirth.

OTHER COMMON USES: Rowan berries were successfully used to treat scurvy as they are rich in vitamins A and C.

The berries ripen in October and are tastiest when cooked with other fruits to make jams and jellies.

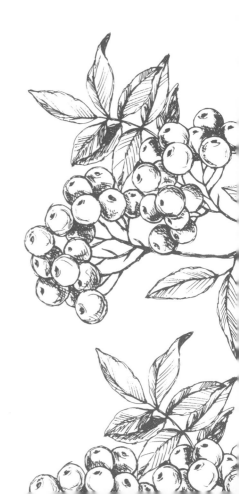

ROWAN BERRY JELLY

Rowan berries are full of vitamins, antioxidants and minerals to help keep away those winter colds. This jelly makes the perfect accompaniment to cheese, game, lamb and charcuterie.

Makes approximately one 500 g jar.

INGREDIENTS

450 g ripe (but not squishy) rowan berries

225 g chopped crab apples or cooking apples

Juice of 1 lemon

Approximately 500 g white sugar

Water

METHOD

Put the washed berries and apples into a heavy-bottomed pan.

Add just enough water to cover the fruit.

Gently simmer the fruit for 15–20 minutes, or until you can mash them easily.

Ladle into a suspended jelly bag or muslin and leave to drip overnight. Don't be tempted to squeeze it or the jelly will be cloudy.

For every 600 ml of juice, add 450 g of white sugar to a pan along with the lemon juice.

Bring to a rolling boil for 10–15 minutes until setting point has been reached.

Spoon off and discard any scum that has formed on top and pour into hot, sterilized jars. Tighten the lid securely and label.

Will keep for up to a year.

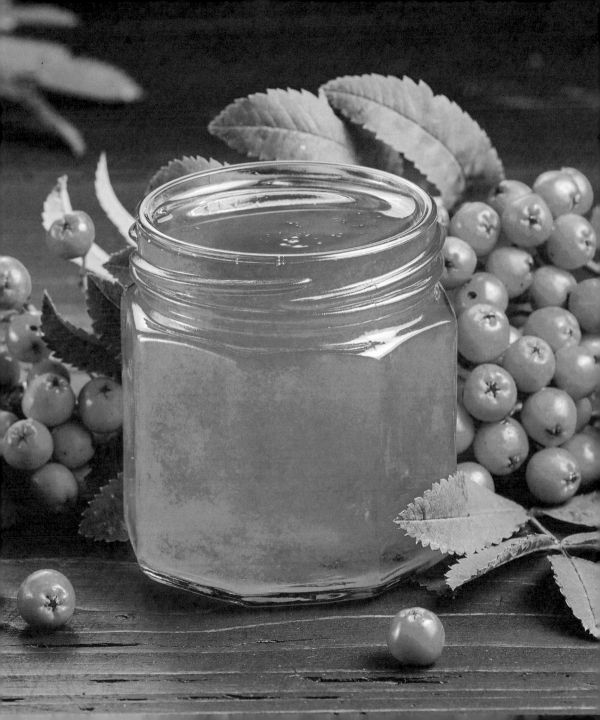

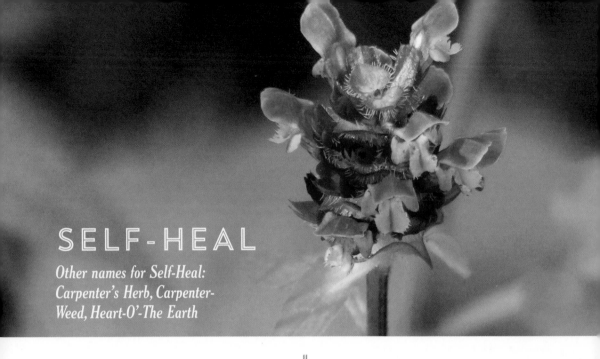

SELF-HEAL

Other names for Self-Heal:
Carpenter's Herb, Carpenter-
Weed, Heart-O'-The Earth

HOW TO IDENTIFY: This low-growing perennial herb is a member of the mint family and can be seen creeping along roadside verges and popping up in untreated lawns. Clusters of small, lip-shaped purple flowers appear on top of square-stemmed spikes from June through to early autumn. It loves damp shady places and is a very important source of nectar for bees and wasps.

HISTORY: Its name tells us that self-heal was a very valuable herb for our ancestors and for all mythical creatures. Prior to World War II, self-heal was used to staunch bleeding and for treating heart disease and cuts and bruises suffered by carpenters. Advances in conventional medicine after the war led to a reduction in the use of natural remedies.

FOLKLORE: Self-heal was valued so highly for healing that children were told never to pick the flower or the devil would come in the dead of night and carry them away – it was far too precious to be picked for pleasure.

Medieval cunning folk and herbalists based some of their treatment on the "Doctrine of Signatures", which taught that if a plant resembled a part of the body, that plant could logically be used to treat any problems that arose with it. So, for example, walnuts were recommended for brain health and tomatoes to treat heart problems.

The tiny flowers of self-heal resemble tiny mouths with swollen glands, the "Signatures" defined its use to be as a remedy for throat complaints.

Druids gathered self-heal at night during the new moon when the Dog Star was rising, as this is when the self-heal was just beginning to bloom. It was dug up with the Druid's golden sickle and then held in the left hand before being split into flowers, leaves and stems to be used in healing magic.

FOLK MEDICINE: This plant has a long history of medicinal use, and traditionally the leaves were applied to wounds to promote healing. According to the sixteenth-century herbalist, John Gerarde:

"there is not a better wounde herb in the world than that of selfheal, the very name importing it to be very admirable."

The seventeenth-century botanist, Nicholas Culpeper, gave the reason for the plant's name as:

"When you are hurt, you may heal yourself."

It was also used to staunch bleeding and to help knit a wound together.

Taken as a tea, it treated fevers, diarrhoea and internal bleeding as well as being used as a gargle for sore throats. The juice was mixed with oil of roses and rubbed on the temples to relieve headaches.

An infusion was often sprayed in the room of a sick person to keep visitors safe from infection.

OTHER COMMON USES: Through a series of modern clinical trials and studies, self-heal has been found to have powerful antiviral properties that combat coughs, colds and fever symptoms. It is effective against a range of bacteria including the one that causes tuberculosis.

No wonder children were discouraged from picking it. What an extraordinary little plant.

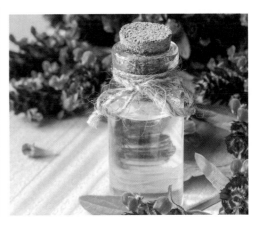

SELF-HEAL PRICKLY HEAT OINTMENT

This wonderful, soothing ointment comes in handy to ease irritation from prickly heat, cooling the affected part of the body

Makes approximately 150 ml.

INGREDIENTS

A large handful of self-heal leaves and flowers

100 ml carrier oil

15 g pure beeswax

METHOD

Place the self-heal in a saucepan and cover with the carrier oil. Warm gently for an hour, allowing the herb to infuse.

Strain through a muslin cloth and squeeze gently to extract every drop of oil.

Put the oil back into the saucepan, add the beeswax and stir over a low heat until the beeswax has melted. Then pour into a dry sterilized jar and allow to cool before popping the lid on.

Should keep in the fridge for up to six months.

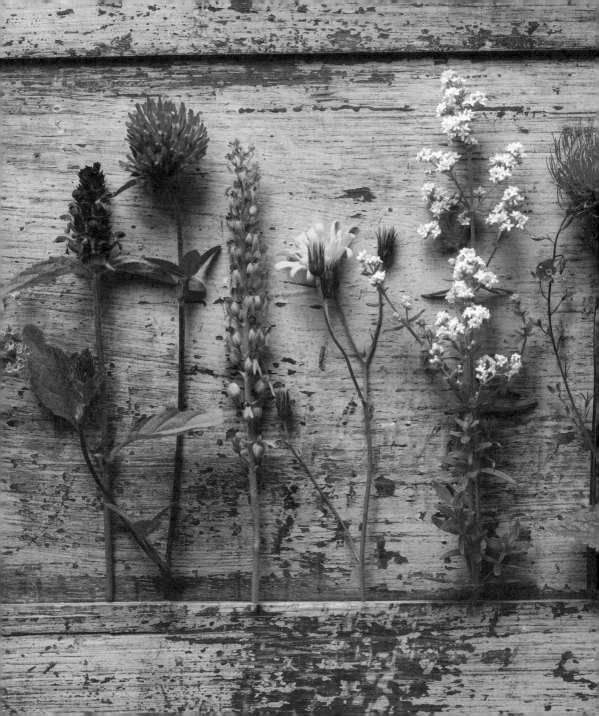

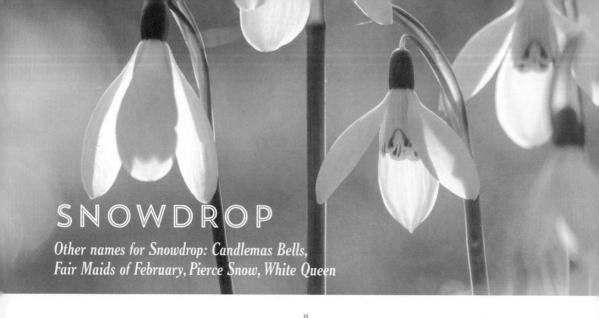

SNOWDROP

Other names for Snowdrop: Candlemas Bells,
Fair Maids of February, Pierce Snow, White Queen

HOW TO IDENTIFY: One of the first wildflowers to appear each year, the snowdrop signals the beginning of spring. Snowdrops have narrow, linear leaves and a straight, flowering stem topped with a single, bell-shaped white flower. Inside each bell are inner petals that have a notch in the tip and a green upside down "V" pattern.

HISTORY: Not native to Britain, snowdrop bulbs were brought over by Italian monks who planted them in monastery gardens.

An old Christian tale tells of how Eve was sad after being banished from the Garden of Eden for her misdemeanours with Adam. Their new home was barren with nothing but heavy snow covering the earth. An angel took pity on her and breathed onto the falling snowflakes, transforming them into white snowdrop flowers, adding just a touch of green to let Eve know that spring was on its way.

FOLKLORE: Although snowdrops were a symbol of hope to Eve, it was considered bad luck to bring them indoors or there would surely be a death before the snowdrops bloomed again. It was safe to grow them in the garden or in pots, but unlucky for the lady of the house to bring them in as her first brood of chickens would not hatch if she did.

According to Laurence Gomme's *The Handbook of Folklore*, published in 1890, it was a common belief that:

"Snowdrops may not be brought in at all, as they will make the cows' milk watery and affect the colour of the butter."

The nodding flowers resemble a corpse in its shroud and because they grow low to the ground and often in churchyards, they were believed to be more connected to the dead than to the living. Snowdrops bloom in February and it was also customary to plant snowdrops on the graves of family members who had died in that month.

Snowdrops should always be picked before St Valentine's Day to ensure that you would get married within the year.

Thought of as shy flowers that are afraid to raise their heads, they actually droop over to keep their dusty pollen dry in the foul wind, rain and snow that come in February.

FOLK MEDICINE: Snowdrops are poisonous to eat and the bulbs have been mistaken for wild garlic or spring onions with fatal consequences.

Early herbalists didn't use snowdrops as they weren't aware of any beneficial properties. Modern research has shown them to be effective as a painkiller for headaches and a compound in the bulb is being developed as a treatment for dementia.

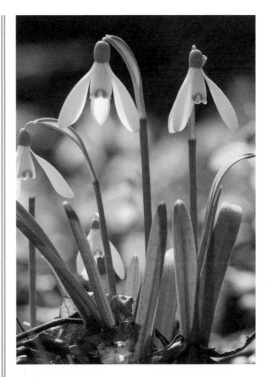

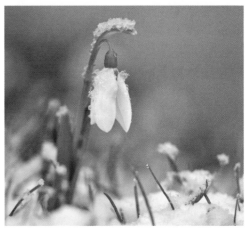

CHEWY LEMON SNOWDROP BISCUITS

A very loosely associated snowdrop recipe, but what a good excuse to stay inside on a cold February day and bake these delicious biscuits!

Makes approximately 20 biscuits.

INGREDIENTS

125 g unsalted butter at room temperature

125 g caster sugar

Grated zest of 1 unwaxed lemon

3 tbsp lemon juice

2 tbsp honey

1 tsp vanilla extract

250 g plain flour

1 tsp baking powder

Pinch of salt

Icing sugar to dust

METHOD

Cream together the butter and sugar until light and fluffy.

Add the lemon zest, lemon juice, honey and vanilla. The mixture may curdle slightly but don't worry. Beat until combined.

Add the flour, baking powder and salt and beat until it forms a stiff dough.

Chill the dough in the fridge for at least 30 minutes.

Preheat oven to 180°C (350°F).

Roll your cold dough into ping-pong-ball-sized pieces and place on an ungreased baking tray, leaving a space between each one.

Bake for 8–10 minutes until the undersides of the biscuits are golden brown.

Allow to cool slightly, then carefully transfer them onto a wire cooling rack.

Once they are completely cold, tumble them in icing sugar and enjoy.

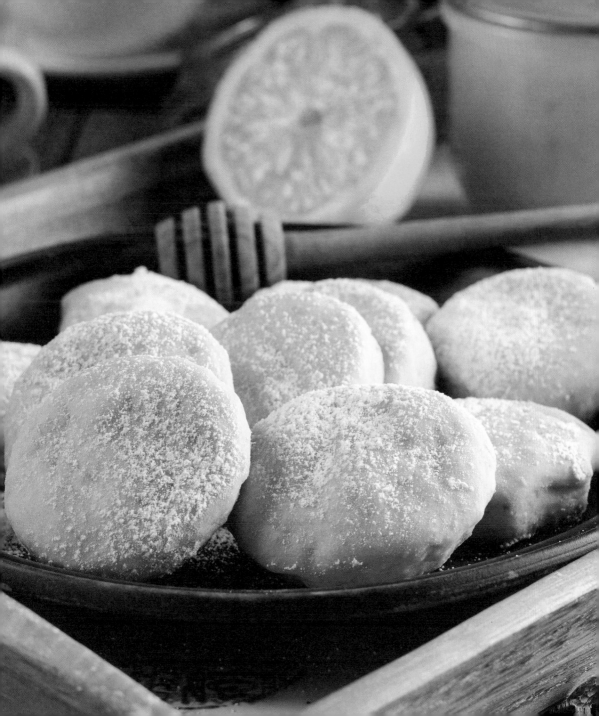

ST JOHN'S WORT

Other names for St John's Wort:
Scare-Devil, Penny John, Goat Weed,
Balm of the Warrior's Wound

HOW TO IDENTIFY: You can find many different species of this lovely plant along the June hedgerow. The bright yellow, star-shaped flowers bloom all summer long. The leaves are easily recognizable as they are about 1.5 cm (half an inch) long and have a perforated appearance: these are actually oil glands, not holes. It grows to about 1 metre (3 feet) tall and readily self-seeds.

This plant blooms during the summer solstice and is believed to be at its most powerful when the sun is at its peak on 24 June, which is St John's Day.

HISTORY: This beautiful plant has always been associated with the power of good. Pagans used it to help celebrate the summer solstice on 21 June. With the coming of Christianity, it was decided to hijack the pagan festival and turn it into the Christian feast day of St John the Baptist.

FOLKLORE: Witches were particularly active on the eve of the festival of St John. The herb was hung over windows and doors to ensure the safety of people, cattle and crops.

Some sound advice from an anonymous poem written in the fourteenth century:

"St John's Wort doth charm
all the witches away
If gathered at midnight on
the saint's holy day
And devils and witches have
no power to harm
Those that do gather the plant for a charm
Rub the lintels and the post
with that red juicy flower
No thunder no tempest will
then have the power
To hurt or hinder your house; and bind
Round your neck a charm of similar kind."

According to the charmingly titled book, *Brand's Popular Antiquities of Great Britain: Faiths and Folklore; a Dictionary of National Beliefs, Superstitions and Popular Customs, Past and Current, with Their Classical and Foreign Analogues, Described and Illustrated, Volume 1*:

> *"If looking for a husband, collect a sprig wet with dew on St John's Day and you will marry within the next year."*

The plant has magical powers and can be used for divination but gathering the flowers can be difficult as the plant sometimes "moves away" from anyone who is trying to pick it. If you are careless enough to step on a flower during the day, faeries will whisk you away on a wild ride across the countryside and then drop you in a ditch, miles from anywhere. Stepping on a flower just before bedtime will ensure that you are kept awake all night by mischievous elves, but to ensure a good night's sleep with no bad dreams, place a sprig of the plant along with some thyme under your pillow.

FOLK MEDICINE: In medieval times, St John's Wort was used in exorcisms to drive out the inner devil, cure hallucinations and as an antidepressant. The "Doctrine of Signatures" was a medieval belief that each plant was put on the Earth to heal and it resembled the part of the body that it could help, for example, eyebright for eye health, walnuts for brain health, and so on. The holes in the leaves of St John's Wort resemble wounds, so it follows that it will be an effective wound healer.

Hold a leaf up to the sunshine and you will clearly see lots of perforations supposedly put there with a needle by the devil in an attempt to destroy this powerful healing herb.

As Culpeper wrote:

> *"It is a singular wound herb, boiled in wine and drank, it heals inward hurts and bruises, made into an ointment, it opens obstructions, dissolves swellings and closes up the lips of wounds."*

Also used as a cure for infertility, gathered naked on Midsummer's Day, you are sure to be pregnant within the year.

OTHER COMMON USES: St John's Wort is still used by herbalists to help treat seasonal affective disorder (SAD) and the darkness of depression. It is also used as a treatment for shingles as it is antiviral and has pain-relieving qualities too.

Not to be used during pregnancy or with medication, including the contraceptive pill.

ST JOHN'S WORT HEALING SALVE

This relaxing massage oil can help to ease sore muscles, sprains, bruises and shingles. To get maximum power from this oil, pick your flowers on Midsummer's Day, but only if the weather is dry.

INGREDIENTS

Flowering tops of St John's Wort

Carrier oil of your choice (almond oil or olive oil, for example)

METHOD

Fill a clean glass jar with the flowers.

Pour in enough oil to completely cover, pop on the lid and shake to release any bubbles. Place on a sunny windowsill.

Shake every now and then, checking that the flowers are submerged.

The oil will turn a beautiful scarlet red.

After a month, strain out the flowers, then bottle and label the oil.

This oil can be used as is or made into a balm by dissolving 1 tsp of beeswax gently into 50 ml of your warmed infused oil. Use within six months.

Be careful, this oil could make your skin more sensitive to the sun.

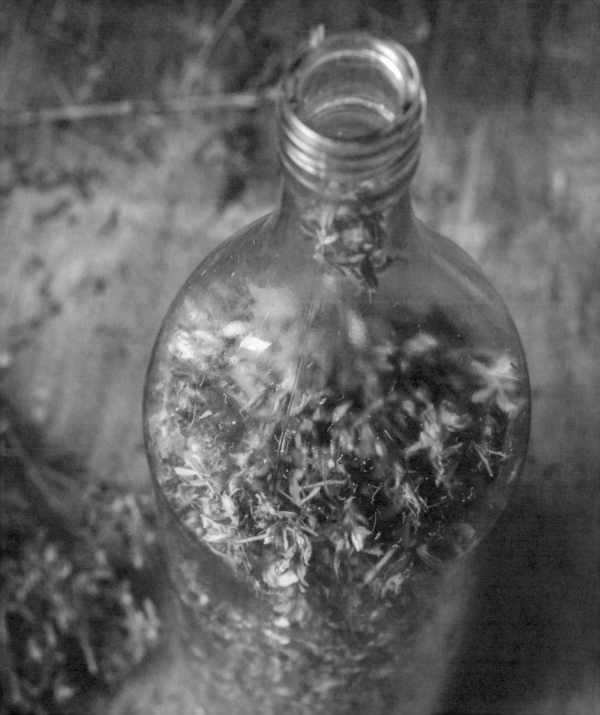

TANSY

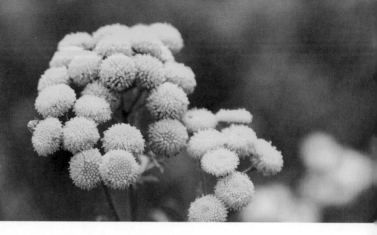

Other names for Tansy:
Bachelor's Buttons, Cow Bitter,
Scented Daisies, Bitter Buttons

HOW TO IDENTIFY: This tall, rather unpleasant-smelling plant can be found on roadside verges and rough grassland. Its fern-like leaves alternate along the straight reddish stem, which is topped in summer by clusters of yellow button flowers, known as "disc florets". These attract lots of insects, especially the endangered tansy beetle that lays its eggs on the flowers and feeds on the leaves.

HISTORY: Although not native to Britain, it was believed that tansy was brought over from Europe to be cultivated for medicinal use. When gathered in Midsummer, the flower heads can keep their colour for months. Tansy was used as a "strewing" herb along with sage, violets, roses, mints, pennyroyal, winter savory, marjoram, hops, germander, sweet fennel, cowslips, lady's mantle, balm, basil, costmary, lavender, juniper, rosemary, chamomile, daisies of all sorts, lavender cotton and sweet woodruff. These aromatic herbs were used to keep mice and insects away, and to make medieval houses smell a little more pleasant. Blacksmiths rubbed tansy into their horses' coats as an insect repellent and to give them a lovely shine. Meat was massaged with tansy leaves to keep flies away, and tansy was often placed in coffins to deter worms and make the dead immortal. Tansy was also called "bible leaf" as it was common to use the leaves as bookmarks in the bible.

FOLKLORE: Tansy cakes are traditionally eaten at Easter to purify the body after the limited diet of Lent. It was customary in some parts of Britain for the local vicar to play a form of "handball" with his congregation, the winners were rewarded with tansy cakes made from eggs and young tansy leaves.

This seventeenth-century tansy recipe was written by Robert May in his book, *The Accomplisht Cook*, first published in 1660:

> *"To make a Tansie the best way.*
> *Take twenty eggs, and take away five*
> *whites, strain them with a quart of good*
> *thick sweet cream, and put to it grated*
> *nutmeg, a race of ginger grated, as much*
> *cinamon beaten fine, and a penny white*
> *loaf grated also, mix them all together*
> *with a little salt, then stamp some green*
> *wheat with some tansie herbs, strain it*
> *into the cream and eggs, and stir all*
> *together; then take a clean frying-pan,*
> *and a quarter of a pound of butter,*
> *melt it, and put in the tansie, and*
> *stir it continually over the fire with*
> *a slice, ladle, or saucer, chop it, and*
> *break it as it thickens, and being well*
> *incorporated put it out of the pan into a*
> *dish, and chop it very fine; then make*
> *the frying pan very clean, and put in*
> *some more butter, melt it, and fry it*
> *whole or in spoonfuls; being finely fried*
> *on both sides, dish it up, and sprinkle*
> *it with rose-vinegar, grape-verjuyce,*
> *elder-vinegar, couslip-vinegar, or the*
> *juyce of three or four oranges, and*
> *strew on good store of fine sugar."*

FOLK MEDICINE: Tansy was used as an infusion to rid humans and animals from intestinal worms. Headlice could also be treated externally with the infusion.

An early twentieth-century manuscript based on dialogue recommends:

"Cure for threadworm – boil the flowers or foliage of tansy weed and drink the infusion. Dose – a wineglass full each morning."

Caution: Today tansy is NOT recommended to be ingested by anyone!

Rabbits, known for their fertility, loved to eat tansy leaves, so it followed that couples wishing to start a family should include tansy in their salads.

In Sussex, tansy leaves were placed into shoes to prevent fevers and the tea, according to Culpeper:

> *"Is also very profitable to dispel wind*
> *in the stomach, belly or bowels."*

This versatile herb was also valuable in the treatment of insomnia, bronchitis, neuralgia, migraine, rheumatism and gout.

OTHER COMMON USES: Bunches of tansy placed on windowsills will deter flies and insects from entering.

INSECT DETERRENT PILLOW

Pop one of these into your linen drawer or hang in your wardrobe to keep moths and other insects away. Hang garden herbs up in a cool, dark place to dry until crumbly or, alternatively, simply buy ready-dried herbs.

INGREDIENTS

Tansy*

Lavender

Thyme

Peppermint

Lemongrass

Cedar chips

Muslin or organza drawstring bag

METHOD

Mix all the herbs together and put into the drawstring bag. Pop into your drawer or wardrobe, remembering to give it a little squeeze occasionally to release the scent.

*Do not use tansy during pregnancy.

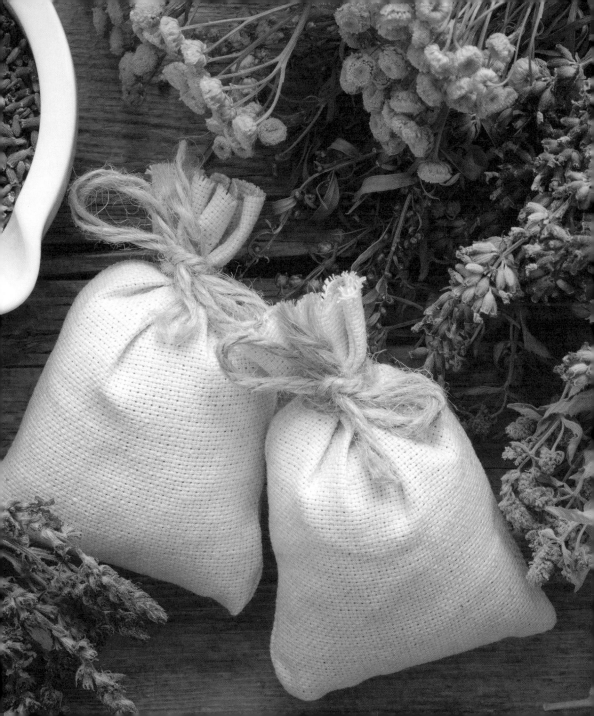

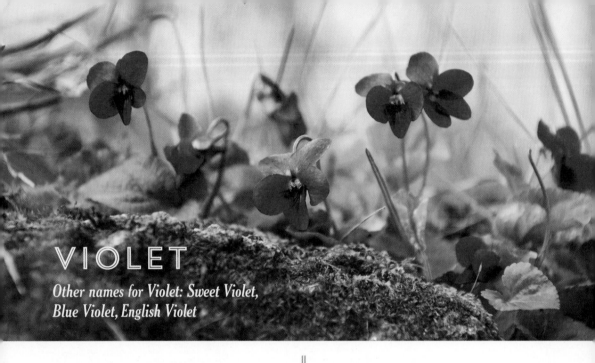

VIOLET

Other names for Violet: Sweet Violet,
Blue Violet, English Violet

HOW TO IDENTIFY: Violets grow on shaded banks, under hedges and in woodland. The pansy-like flowers appear from late March to early April and are not always violet in colour, but can be white, pink or dark indigo blue. When eaten, they have a faint taste of Parma Violets sweets. The heart-shaped leaves are slightly downy and start off bright green, turning darker as they age.

HISTORY: Violets were particularly popular in the medieval era. These flowers were used to perfume linens and potpourri, and to flavour meads and alcoholic drinks. Violets were also added to both sweet and savoury dishes. Monks grew violet lawns to give them somewhere fragrant to sit and meditate. The violet was one of Queen Victoria's favourite flowers and was sold on the streets of London, as well as being used extensively in the perfume industry at the time. Known as a plant to symbolize fidelity, the poet William Hunnis wrote:

> *"Violet is for faithfulness,*
> *Which in me shall abide.*
> *Hoping likewise that from your heart,*
> *You will not let it slide."*

It was believed that the violet was present at the crucifixion and hangs its sweet head in mourning. This association with death, especially the death of a young person, is reinforced by Shakespeare when writing of Ophelia:

"Lay her in the earth; And from her fair and unpolluted flesh may violets spring!"

FOLKLORE: Dreaming of violets is said to predict prosperity, and an infusion of violets in hot water can be taken to aid sleep and also to soothe anger. The Romans and Greeks believed that wearing a crown of violets would protect them from the effects of too much alcohol.

The English botanist, Reverend John Lightfoot, wrote in 1777 that some people in Scotland recommended violets and goat's milk to women seeking flawless skin:

"Anoint thy face with goat's milk in which violets have been infused and there is not a young prince on earth who would not be charmed by thy beauty."

In *The Diary of a Farmer's Wife 1796–1797* by Anne Hughes, it is instructed that a good cure for a grouchy husband is to serve him violet pudding.

I have discovered that folkloric advice is often contradictory, and violets are a prime example of this. Violets generally flower around the spring equinox, when they should be picked, dried and kept as an amulet to protect against evil spirits. However, folklore also warns not to bring violets into the house as they are associated with death, attract fleas and are likely to keep your chickens off the lay.

FOLK MEDICINE: In 1653, Culpeper writes of his rather unusual remedy for haemorrhoids using violets fried with eggs and applied to the offending area. The leaves were also used as a gentle laxative called "violet plate" for children.

In the 1930s, *The Woman's Treasury for Home and Garden* by A. J. Macself, published this recipe for violet cough syrup:

"Pick the petals from their calyces (sepals) and use one ounce. Boil for 5 minutes in a pint of water with 8 ounces of sugar. Strain through muslin, bottle and use in one-teaspoon doses as occasion demands."

The sweet scent of violets was used to treat headaches and insomnia and to help cheer you up and heal wounds.

OTHER COMMON USES: Still used in sweets and chocolates as well as perfumes, soaps and cosmetics, and sewn into small pillows to aid a good night's sleep.

CRYSTALLIZED VIOLET FLOWERS

Other edible flowers such as pansies, borage and rose petals can be crystallized along with violets to create beautiful decorations for cakes and biscuits. Violets are easily cultivated and spread quickly, so rather than pick from the wild, why not grow a small patch of edible flowers such as heartsease, borage, nasturtiums and violets? The bees will appreciate them too.

INGREDIENTS

Freshly picked
violet flowers

Egg white

Caster sugar

METHOD

Whisk the egg white lightly, just enough to break down the albumin.

Using a fine brush, paint the front and back of the flowers with egg white,* making sure that all areas are covered.

Sprinkle sugar all over the flowers, shaking off the excess, and place them face down on baking paper.

The flowers need to dry uncovered for at least 24 hours, longer if the flowers are thicker.

Store in an airtight container and use within a couple of days.

*For a vegan alternative, simply paint the leaves with aquafaba (chickpea liquid) instead of egg white.

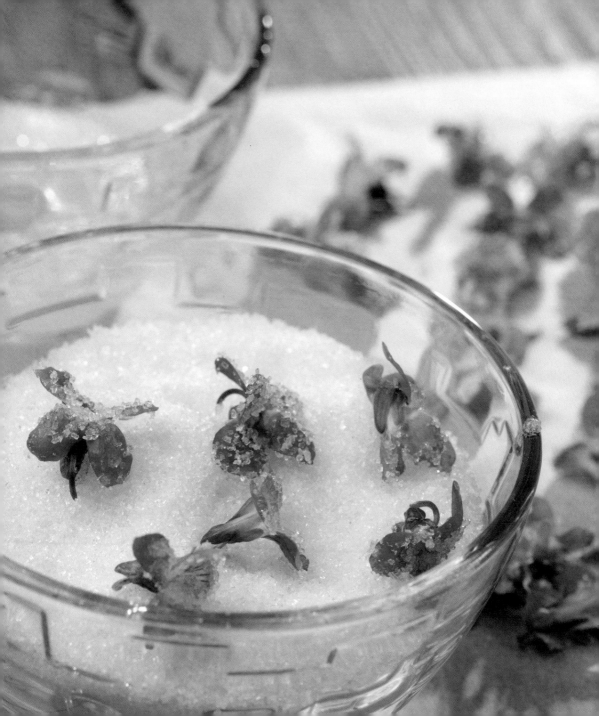

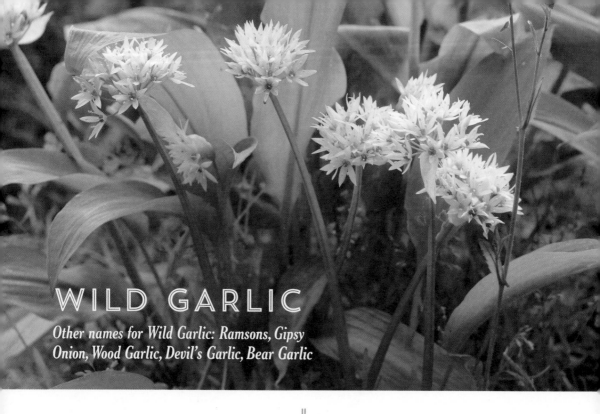

WILD GARLIC

Other names for Wild Garlic: Ramsons, Gipsy Onion, Wood Garlic, Devil's Garlic, Bear Garlic

HOW TO IDENTIFY: Wild garlic grows in damp, ancient woodlands and has a very distinctive, garlicky smell. Be careful when foraging for wild garlic as the leaves look very similar to both lily of the valley and lords and ladies, which are poisonous. Crush the leaves and sniff them for that pungent garlic smell. Its broad, spear-like leaves appear in early March, followed by a profusion of starry white flowers carpeting the woodland floor. Leaves, bulbs and flowers are all edible, adding a subtle garlic flavour to food.

HISTORY: Wild garlic leaves have often been used as fodder, and cows that are fed on the leaves produce milk with a slightly garlicky flavour, which is lovely for garlic butter.

Wild garlic, along with wood anemone, wood spurge, small-leaved lime and guelder rose, are all indicators of ancient woodland. The wild garlic you forage may well have been gathered in the same place by our ancestors hundreds of years ago. It is illegal to dig up the bulbs, but it is permitted to gather the leaves with the consent of the landowner.

FOLKLORE: The plant's common name of "bear garlic" comes from the belief that bears – as well as wild boar and badgers – ate wild garlic to regain their strength after a winter of hibernation.

Wild garlic was planted in the thatch of Irish cottages to ward off faeries and bring good luck. Soldiers heading to battle and athletes about to compete chewed a piece of wild garlic to give them strength for victory.

FOLK MEDICINE: With all the same medicinal benefits of cultivated garlic – high in antioxidants, immune-boosting powers and so on – it's no wonder that this magical plant was so valuable to our ancestors. Wild garlic cleanses the blood and intestines, improves the intestinal flora and helps with acne and eczema, as well as boosting the body's immune system. It can be made into poultices to treat bad knees and mixed with lard and rubbed into the soles of feet as a treatment for bronchitis. The plant is said to be a "cure all". An infusion was drunk to strengthen the blood, infected wounds could be cured by a poultice and the strong smell of the leaves was used to repel insects.

Culpeper says of wild garlic:

"It wonderfully opens the lungs, and gives relief to asthmas, and is a good diuretic."

In the spring, the bulbs can be dug up, covered in dark brown sugar and rum, and then left until the winter to be used as a remedy for coughs and colds.

Many people in Ireland carried ramsons in their pockets to guard against flu during the epidemic of 1918.

Romany gypsies are known to call it "the fountain of youth".

OTHER COMMON USES: Similar in taste to chives, the young, tender leaves can be used in salads and sauces, added to scrambled eggs or omelettes, stirred into risottos, or my favourite way to use them – pesto.

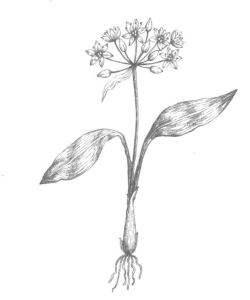

WILD GARLIC PESTO

Pesto is pretty much raw when eaten, keeping all the valuable antiviral, antibiotic and antibacterial properties and vitamins intact. Pick young, tender garlic leaves away from busy roads and dog-walkers. It should be picked before the flowers appear, as once they do, the leaves become tough and leathery and are not really worth picking.

INGREDIENTS

Handful of well-washed young wild garlic leaves

Handful of basil leaves

200 g finely grated parmesan cheese

150 g pine nuts (or walnuts)

Olive oil

Salt to taste

METHOD

Blend the wild garlic and basil in a pestle and mortar or food processor with enough olive oil to make a smooth paste.

Stir in the parmesan cheese and roughly chopped nuts. Season to taste.

Stir through freshly cooked pasta, knead into bread dough or slip under the skin of a chicken before roasting.

Store in the fridge and use within 3 days.

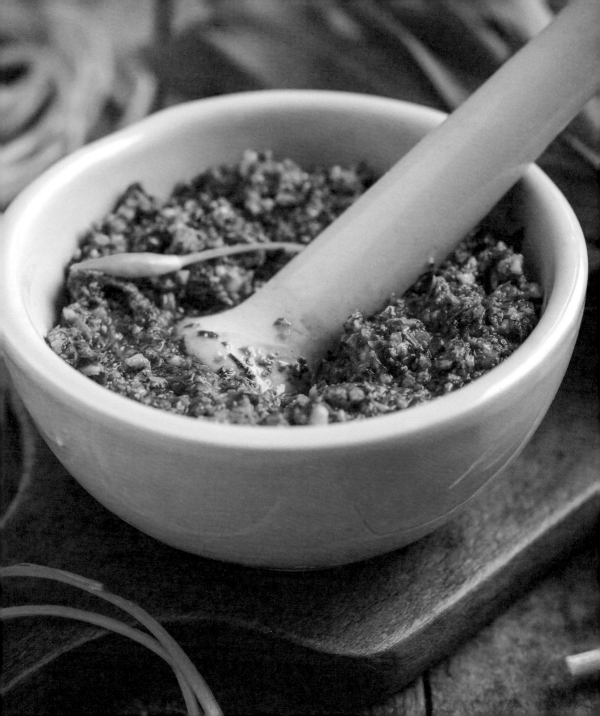

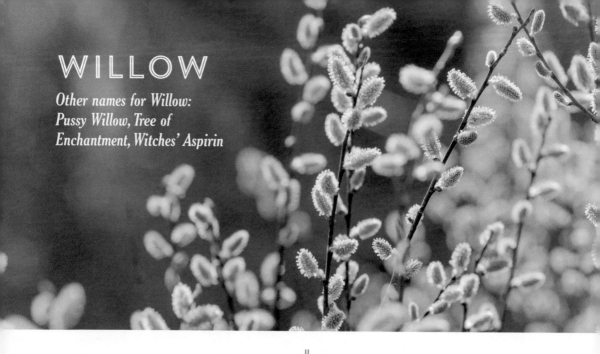

WILLOW

Other names for Willow:
Pussy Willow, Tree of
Enchantment, Witches' Aspirin

HOW TO IDENTIFY: Willow is a tall, deciduous tree with grey/brown bark that develops deep cracks over time. The twigs are long, slender and very flexible, making them useful for various crafts. Willow can be found along river banks, in wet woodlands, and around lakes. Long yellow catkins appear in spring, providing much-needed nectar for insects that, in return, pollinate the tree. The slender, oval-shaped leaves are covered on the underside with silky hairs, which make them appear white as the wind tumbles them.

HISTORY: In 1763, after much experimentation, Reverend Edward Stone discovered that willow bark was effective in reducing fevers in his parishioners. It wasn't until 1853 that the French scientist, Charles Gerhardt, successfully made a primitive form of aspirin that went on to be marketed to the public in 1899, and the synthesized version is almost certainly one of the most-used drugs in the world today.

FOLKLORE: Willow wands are used in magic mainly for healing spells and were given as gifts of friendship, love and good luck at Beltane (May Day).

Young ladies, who wished to find out who they were to marry, would run three times around their houses carrying the willow wand. It is said an image of their future husband would appear holding the other end of the wand.

The flexible shoots were employed to bind the twigs onto witches' brooms. It is thought that the term "Wicca" (witchcraft) came from "wicker" – the common name for willow twigs.

Also known as a tree of sadness and mourning, "wearing the willow" meant the wearer was openly grieving either for a dead loved one or a lost love.

In ancient Greece, it was common for willow twigs to be laid in, and on top of, coffins to help the soul depart safely:

"Plant as willow and allow it to grow,
To ease the passage of your soul at death."

Celts planted willow saplings on graves in the belief that the essential nature of the departed person would be preserved in that tree.

Knocking on wood for luck is a commonly known superstition; willow should be used if possible, as it will bring you luck and also ward off the evil eye.

Never beat your child with a willow twig or they will not grow from that moment on.

FOLK MEDICINE: Culpeper clearly held the willow in high regard as he wrote:

"Both the leaves, bark, and the seed,
are used to staunch bleeding of wounds,
and at mouth and nose, spitting of
blood, and other fluxes of blood in man
or woman, and to stay vomiting."

Because the willow grows in wet places, it followed that it must offer protection against "damp" ailments such as rheumatism. It was keenly sought out by old crones who came to the tree by the light of the moon seeking a cure.

The seeds drunk in spring water were used as an aphrodisiac by men, although the downside was that they would only father barren daughters and no sons.

OTHER COMMON USES: Many uses for willow include: wicker baskets, willow screens, shelters and sculptures, woven fences and charcoal.

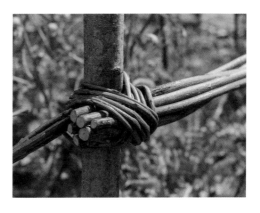

WILLOW BARK SALVE

A lovely salve to massage into sore muscles or relieve the pain of arthritis in joints using the natural painkiller found in willow. As well as smelling wonderful, lavender oil and calendula are both anti-inflammatory and analgesic.

INGREDIENTS

100 ml carrier oil

50 g dried willow bark (available online)

10 g dried lavender flowers

10 g dried calendula flowers

10 drops of lavender essential oil

10 g natural beeswax

METHOD

Using a double boiler or heatproof bowl over a pan of water, pour in the carrier oil along with all of the dried herbs. Warm gently for 2–3 hours – the longer you warm it, the more infused it will become.

Strain the infused oil into a clean jug and then back into the double boiler for the next stage.

Begin to warm the oil gently and add the lavender essential oil and beeswax until it has just melted; watch carefully, and don't allow the mixture to boil.

Pour into clean, dry containers, allowing to cool before popping on the lid.

Keep in the fridge to maintain freshness and use as needed.

Not to be used during pregnancy or if allergic to aspirin.

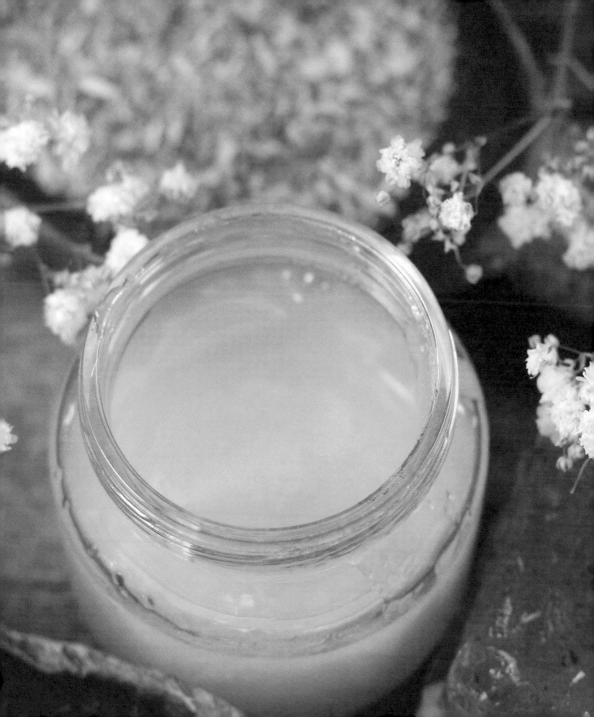

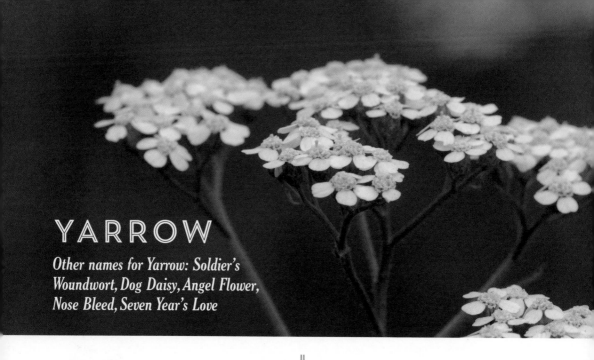

YARROW

Other names for Yarrow: Soldier's Woundwort, Dog Daisy, Angel Flower, Nose Bleed, Seven Year's Love

HOW TO IDENTIFY: Yarrow is found in abundance in grassland all over Britain. This ferny leaved perennial can grow up to 1 metre (3 feet) tall. The plant forms clumps that can be quite invasive with long, straight stalks and feathery leaves, with white or pink flowers at the top.

Crush the leaves and you will release its strong aromatic smell.

HISTORY: Our Anglo-Saxon ancestors had great respect for yarrow due to its powerful wound-healing properties. In the Middle Ages, before the widespread use of hops, yarrow was one of the many herbs used along with bog myrtle and wild rosemary to make *"gruit"* – an early form of beer.

FOLKLORE: Unmarried maidens in medieval Sussex would pick yarrow from a young man's grave by the light of the full moon and put it under their pillow saying:

> *"Good night fair yarrow,*
> *Thrice goodnight to thee,*
> *I hope before tomorrow,*
> *My true love to see."*

They would also pin it to their dresses and get as close to their potential suitors as possible. When they got home, the yarrow was placed in a drawer, if it was still fresh the next morning their love would be reciprocated.

Often known as "seven year's love", yarrow was included in bridal bouquets, hung over the marriage bed and often eaten at wedding breakfasts to ensure that the couple were happy for at least seven years.

Yarrow tea was used by witches to enhance their psychic powers and holding the plant up to the eyes gives the power of second sight.

FOLK MEDICINE: Yarrow has been used as a remedy for many ailments. The dark blue essential oil from the flowers is a good chest rub for colds and flu, the leaves encourage clotting and can be used for nosebleeds. Leaves, stems and flowers are used to stimulate the circulation, lower blood pressure and as a tonic for the blood.

An infusion of yarrow applied to the scalp will prevent baldness but unfortunately won't be able to cure it. Also used as a treatment for snakebites, a cure for colds and flu, a tea to help insomnia and give relief from toothache. Headaches were believed to be caused by too much blood pressure in the head; yarrow leaves were pushed up the nostrils to cause bleeding to ease the pressure.

Gerarde, in his *The Herball or Generall Historie of Plantes* (1597), states that:

> *"The leaves being put into the nose do cause it to bleed, and easeth the pain of the megrin."*

Conversely, smelling yarrow flowers was also believed to be a cure for nosebleeds.

OTHER COMMON USES: Yarrow is a useful herb to hang in your wardrobe as it deters insects. Yarrow was a popular vegetable in the seventeenth century; the young leaves were cooked like spinach or put into soup. The leaves can also be dried and used as a cooking herb.

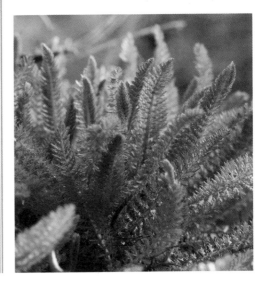

YARROW AND CALENDULA HARMONY TEA

This lovely tea brings balance and harmony back into the female body. Yarrow and calendula stimulate blood flow to the womb, vervain balances emotions and brings calm, lady's mantle is a diuretic and raspberry leaf helps with period pains.

INGREDIENTS

1 tsp yarrow

1 tsp calendula flowers

1 tsp lady's mantle
(available online)

1 tsp vervain

1 tsp raspberry leaf

METHOD

Place all the ingredients into a jug then pour over 500 ml of boiling water.

Cover and allow it to infuse for 10–15 minutes.

Drink hot or cold throughout the day when you feel the symptoms of PMS appear.

Not to be used during pregnancy.

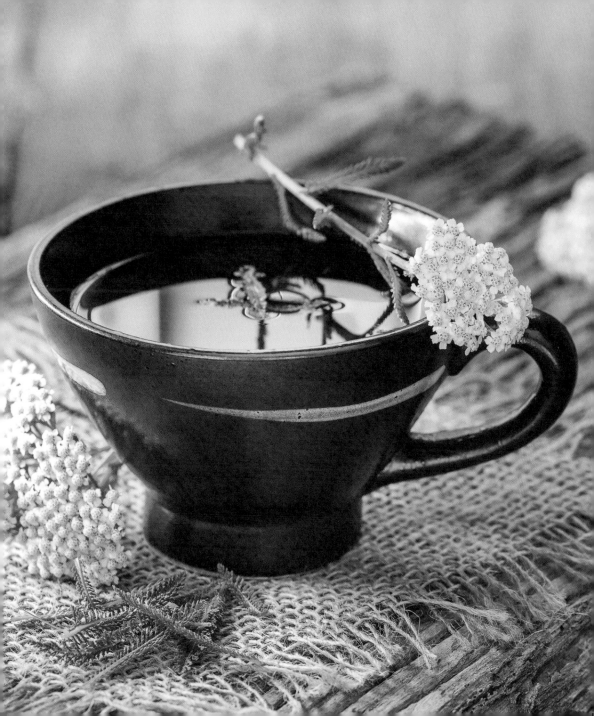

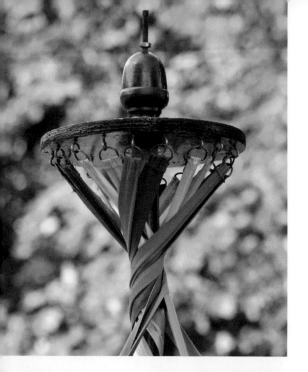

FESTIVALS

The lives of our Celtic forefathers were dominated by "the wheel of the year", which was made up of eight distinct festivals. These dictated to them when the season was right to sow, plough, harvest, celebrate and take some rest. The wheel turns continually according to the position of the sun and represents the never-ending cycle of the birth, death and rebirth of nature. The seasons are still incredibly important as our very existence relies completely on abundant harvests. Even though we can now pretty much eat fruit and vegetables all year round, nothing tastes as delicious as food harvested in season that has been locally sourced or foraged.

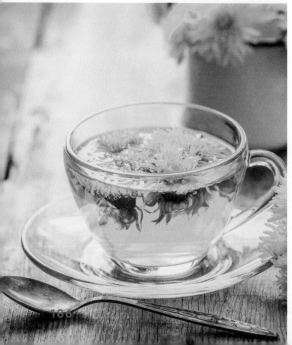

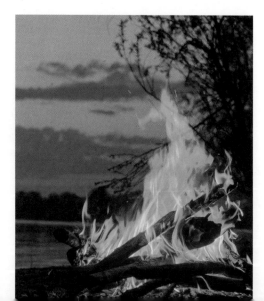

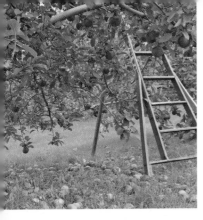
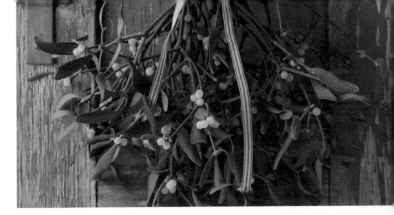
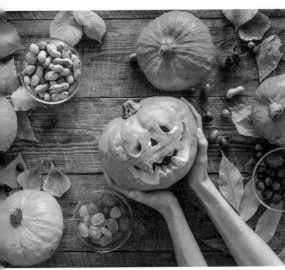
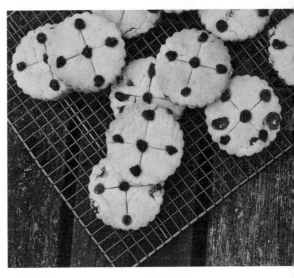
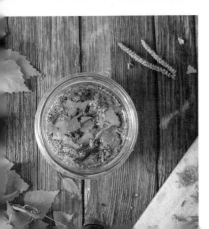
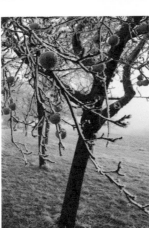
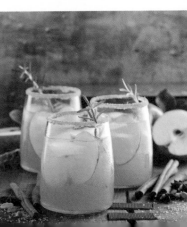

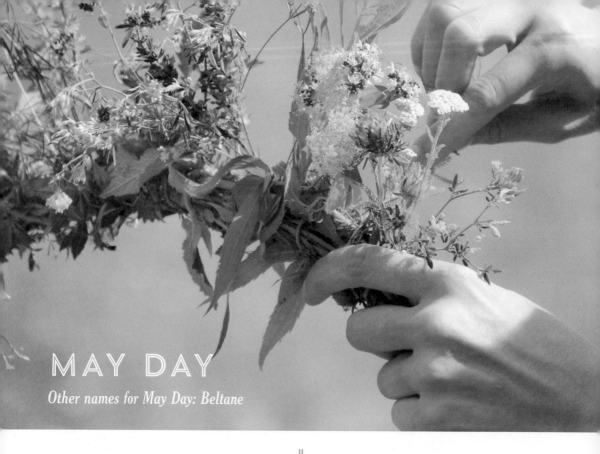

MAY DAY

Other names for May Day: Beltane

This ancient Celtic celebration is known as Beltane from the Celtic word meaning "fires of Bel". It begins on 30 April and continues until 1 May. It is a festival to welcome the coming of summer with anticipation of the abundant fertility of the year. Beltane rituals would often include courting; young couples would collect blossoms in the woods, make love and commit to marriages of a year and a day known as "handfastings". These handfasting ceremonies involved the tying together of hands with a red cord in a figure of eight for the duration of the ceremony, the hands are later untied to symbolize that the union has been entered into with free will. The couple would then "jump the broomstick" to denote moving from their old life to a new one.

Not everyone could afford a church service and many just didn't want one.

Handfasting meant that they could be recognized as a married couple by their community.

Celts lit huge bonfires celebrating the return of light and fertility to the Earth, single men and women would jump over the fire to attract a partner, even pregnant women would jump through the fire to ensure a trouble-free birth.

The origins of the maypole hark back to ancient times when tree spirits were worshipped, and indeed the first maypoles were tall, slender trees, usually birch. These had their branches taken off, leaving just a few at the top to be adorned with garlands and blossom. The finding, decorating and erecting of the village maypole was an important part of community life, becoming the focal point for dancing and merrymaking.

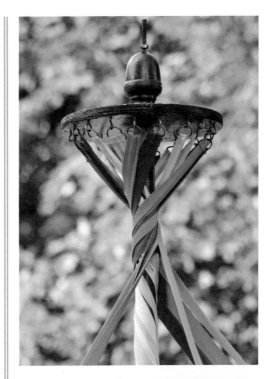

During the Reformation, Puritans became increasingly disapproving of May Day celebrations, especially maypoles, seeing them as immoral and blasphemous. However, after the Reformation, maypoles made a welcome comeback into village life.

May Queens as we know them were reinvented by the Victorians but bear little resemblance to ancient tradition. Historically, a man and a woman, known as "Lord" and "Lady" were chosen by local children to preside over the celebrations.

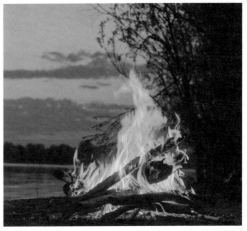

BELTANE DANDELION TONIC

This delicious tonic will refresh the body after a long winter. Full of vitamins A, B12 and C, this sunny little herb spring cleans your body and serves as a reminder that summer isn't too far away.

Makes approximately 1 litre.

INGREDIENTS

Large handful of young dandelion heads* (about 50 g)

1 litre fresh orange juice

Juice of one lemon

Local raw honey, to taste

METHOD

Rinse the dandelion heads in cool water; make sure that you don't have any of the green parts as they are bitter. Warm the orange and lemon juice together, add the dandelion heads and heat without boiling for a further couple of minutes. Strain the juice. Cool slightly before adding honey to taste.

Pop into the fridge and once cold, dilute with still or sparkling mineral water.

Use within one week.

*Always pick your flowers from a pesticide-free and dog-free site.

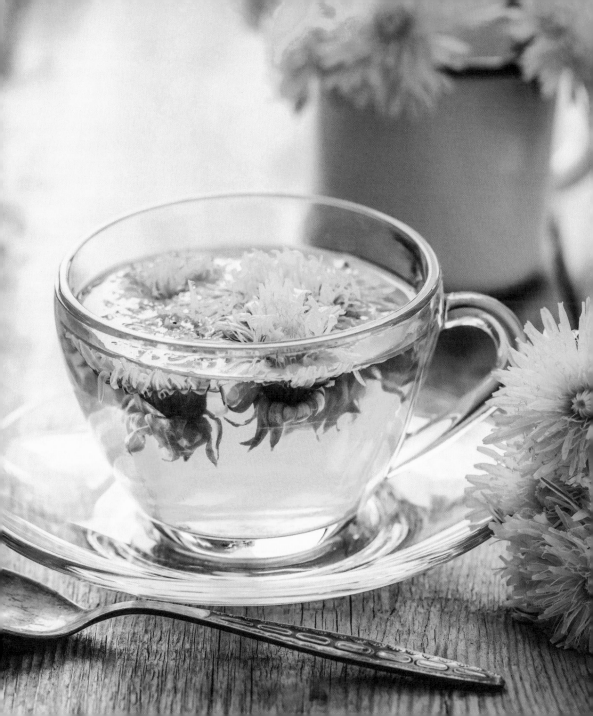

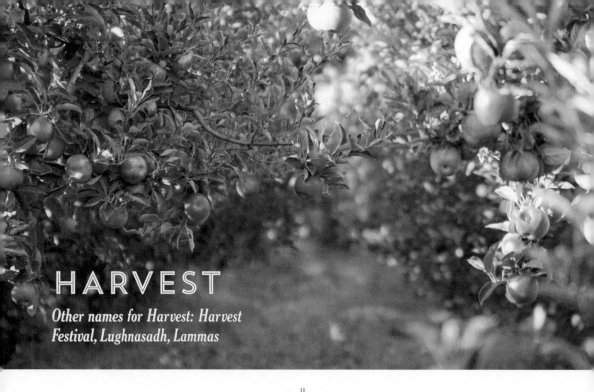

HARVEST

Other names for Harvest: Harvest Festival, Lughnasadh, Lammas

HISTORY: Harvest is one of our oldest known festivals. It is traditionally celebrated in August on the harvest moon or on the full moon that is nearest to the autumn equinox. The word "Lammas" is derived from "Loaf Mass" due to the first grain being harvested that made the first loaf and began the whole harvesting cycle. Lughnasadh, named after the pagan god Lugh, involved village gatherings with ritual ceremonies and much feasting.

It's the season when fruit is ripening, the grain is ready, and we are thankful for the food on our tables.

The success or failure of the crop was an anxious time for our Celtic ancestors, honouring gods and goddesses with a little inducement in the form of the first loaf was vital to ensure the success of the next year's harvest. One Celtic goddess, the Grain Mother, is heavily pregnant with a daughter, Persephone. Persephone signifies the fertile seed that will be placed into the earth; she will sleep all winter and emerge in the springtime, bringing new life with her. Persephone's father is the sun god, Lugh, sometimes called John Barleycorn or the Green Man;

he embodies the spirit of the grain and will surrender his life every Lammas to the harvest when the first corn is cut.

The Scottish poet, Robert Burns, even wrote a poem about the life and death of John Barleycorn:

> *"They took a plough*
> *and plough'd him down,*
> *Put clods upon his head,*
> *And they hae sworn a solemn oath,*
> *John Barleycorn was dead."*

After another eleven verses of trying to kill him, they finally conceded that they could not destroy John Barleycorn as he will, thankfully, re-emerge again every spring.

FOLKLORE: Anglo-Saxon farmers cut the first sheaf of wheat at dawn, removed the chaff, ground the grain into flour and baked the harvest bread. This was to be shared with all the villagers and with Lugh, the god of fertility, at the end of harvest, ensuring a good crop the following year.

The last sheaf was thought to contain the Spirit of the Corn and its cutting was usually accompanied by the ritual sacrifice of an animal; often a hare caught hiding in the corn. The last sheaf would be taken home and made into "corn dollies" to be celebrated at the harvest supper, hung over the fireplace until the next Lammas. The "corn dollies" were a symbol of the Grain Mother and often had a small corn – Persephone – placed inside them.

These traditions continued after Christianity arrived in Britain, though sometimes in a slightly different form. There were ceremonies and rituals at the beginning, as well as the end, of the harvest. The local church would ring its bells on every day that the harvest was being gathered in. The last load to be brought in was celebrated with triumph, usually on a highly decorated wagon with children riding on top.

The most important part of the harvest celebrations was the harvest supper or harvest home. The farmer would provide a magnificent spread for his workers and their families.

In his book, *The Spirit of the Downs. Impressions and Reminiscences of the Sussex Downs* (published in 1909), Arthur Beckett described the celebration as an:

> *"event celebrated for heavy feeding,*
> *curious songs and big drinking feats."*

One last activity in the fields was that the "gleaning bell" would toll and poor women and children were allowed to go "gleaning" to collect any leftover usable crops to help feed their families.

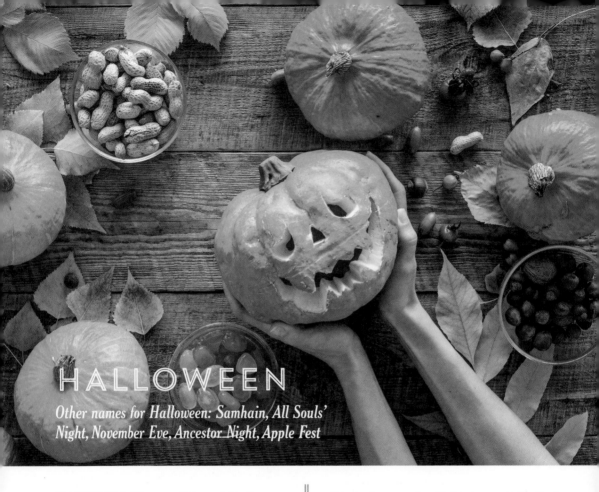

HALLOWEEN

*Other names for Halloween: Samhain, All Souls'
Night, November Eve, Ancestor Night, Apple Fest*

HISTORY: The tradition of Halloween, celebrated on 31 October, is widely believed to have come from America, but it actually originated in Britain. It grew out of the ancient Celtic festival of Samhain, which was one of the major events of "The Wheel of the Year", marking the end of the light half of the year and the beginning of winter.

Samhain was the Celtic harvest festival, when all crops of barley, oats, apples, turnips and wheat must be gathered in. With the arrival of November came the faeries who would blast every growing plant with their freezing breath, ruining all that was left in the fields or hedgerows. With barely enough food to survive the winter, the Celts would have to kill most of their cattle and store the meat as best they could; this meant that Samhain was also a night of great communal feasting.

Halloween started to become Christianized in the Middle Ages in an attempt to blend pagan customs with Christian ones. The date of 1 November became "All Saints' Day", having been moved from 13 May by Pope Gregory III in a deliberate attempt to hijack and disrupt any pagan celebrations.

Bonfires had been important at this time of year and were used by the Celts to burn the harvest chaff and purify the land ready for the next season of growing. Later, bonfires were also seen as a way of helping to guide Christian souls out of purgatory or as a means of protection from witchcraft and the plague.

A tradition that began in the Middle Ages and lasted until around the eighteenth century was "souling", whereby children went from house to house singing rhymes and saying prayers for the dead in return for food. The soul cakes they received as payment for their songs meant that a soul was freed from purgatory and could ascend to heaven, and this was possibly the origin of trick or treating.

In 1891, the Reverend M. P. Holme of Cheshire wrote down this traditional souling song, told to him by a little girl from the local primary school:

"Soul, soul, a soul cake!
I pray thee, good missus, a soul cake!
One for Peter, two for Paul,
Three for Him what made us all!
Soul cake, soul cake, please
good missus, a soul cake."

FOLKLORE: Love divination was very popular on Halloween; young girls, desperate to dream of their future husband, would put a sprig of rosemary and a crooked sixpence under their pillows. Alternatively, they would peel an apple in one continuous strip and throw it over their left shoulder to reveal the initials of their future love.

The custom of carving jack-o'-lanterns goes back to the Irish legend of Jack, a lazy but shrewd farmer who tricked the devil into not sending him to hell. When Jack died, he was too sinful to be allowed into heaven and the devil wouldn't let him into hell. So, Jack carved out one of his turnips, later to become a pumpkin, put a candle inside it and began endlessly wandering Earth for a resting place.

SOUL CAKES

Traditionally given to the poor on Halloween during medieval times, soul cakes were made with sweet spices and dried fruit. These scone-like cakes were marked with the sign of the cross to signify that they were alms to be given to the poor. (Alms are money or food given to poor people as an act of charity.) This is something unusual to hand out to any Halloween trick or treaters, and how satisfying to revive a tradition started by our ancestors!

Makes approximately 12 cakes.

INGREDIENTS

175 g butter

175 g caster sugar

3 free range egg yolks, beaten

450 g plain flour

2 tsp mixed spice

100 g currants

Milk

METHOD

Preheat oven to 190°C (375°F).

Cream the butter and sugar together until light and fluffy, then beat the egg yolks in little by little.

Sieve the flour and spice into the wet mixture. Add most of the currants and stir to combine, but save some of the currants to decorate the tops with. If the mixture is too dry, add a little milk to bring it all together into a soft dough.

On a floured board, roll the dough out to a thickness of approximately 1 cm (³/₈ inch), cut into rounds and place onto a baking sheet lined with baking paper.

Using the back of a knife, mark each cake with the sign of the cross and dot the remaining currants along these lines.

Bake for 10–15 minutes until golden brown.

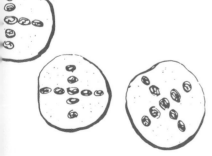

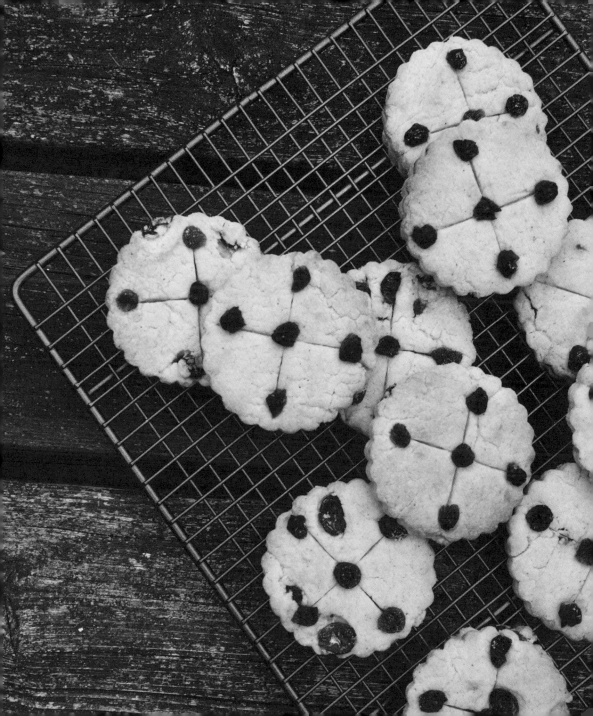

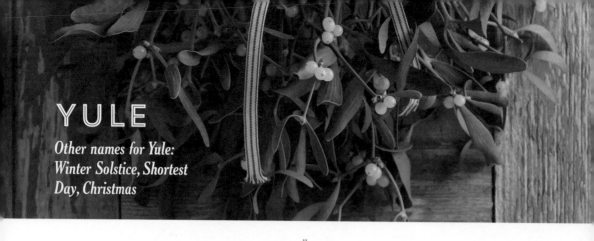

YULE

Other names for Yule:
Winter Solstice, Shortest
Day, Christmas

Yule is traditionally celebrated on the winter solstice, around 21 December, when darkness has reached its peak and daylight hours begin to lengthen. Yule has been marked by Celts in Britain long before the arrival of Christianity. Celtic priests, known as Druids, cut down the mistletoe growing on oak trees with great ceremony using golden scythes. It would be blessed as a symbol of life that was still surviving despite the long dark winter months.

Celtic folklore tells us that the Holly King, who represents the waning year, rules from Midsummer to Yule. At Yule he surrenders to the Oak King, otherwise known as the Sun King, who rules the waxing half of the year from Midwinter to Midsummer. Both surrender their lives at the end of their rule for the good of the land. The Celts thought the sun stood still for twelve days over the Yule period; to conquer the darkness and protect themselves from evil spirits, they dragged a huge oak log into the house to burn. It was decorated with holly, pinecones and ivy, splashed with ale and then lit with a piece of the previous year's Yule log that had been kept especially for the occasion. Once burned, the log's ashes were valuable treasures said to have medicinal and magical powers that were able to guard against evil. It was claimed the ashes would protect the bearer from lightning, which was valuable at a time when houses, and most of the contents in them, were made out of wood.

Until the fourth century, Yule was celebrated by pagans throughout Europe.

Pope Julius I decided to adopt 25 December as the actual date of the birth of Christ. His choice of date was very clever; any pagan merrymaking could now be associated with the birth of Christ rather than to any ancient pagan ritual.

The word "Christmas" had replaced "Yule" in most of England by the eleventh century.

Medieval records show that "villeins" – peasant farmers tied to a manor – were not required to work during the twelve days of Christmas and that the lord of the manor would provide a communal feast.

The tradition of baking Twelfth Night cakes goes back to medieval times when they were an important part of Yule celebrations and were offered to the priest and his clergy as payment for their blessing on the household. Full of dried fruit and expensive spices, these were the forerunners to our traditional Christmas cake.

The earliest printed recipe for Twelfth Cakes appears to have been written in *The Art of Cookery Made Easy and Refined* in 1803 by John Mollard, a prestigious London chef who owned many restaurants from the 1780s through to the 1830s. As you can see, he must have entertained many guests on Twelfth Night:

"Take seven pounds of flour, make a cavity in the centre, set a sponge with a gill and a half of yeast and a little warm milk; then put round it one pound of fresh butter broke into small lumps, one pound and a quarter of sifted sugar, four pounds and a half of currants washed and picked, half an ounce of sifted cinnamon, a quarter of an ounce of powdered cloves, mace, nutmeg and mixed, sliced candied orange or lemon peel and citron. When the sponge is risen, mix all the ingredients together with warm milk; let the hoops be well papered and buttered, then fill them with the mixture and bake them..."

By Tudor times, Christmas at court was celebrated by magnificent banquets, often with a "Lord of Misrule" who would caricature the court alongside an "Abbot of Unreason" who would ridicule the Church. In the sixteenth and seventeenth centuries, Puritans put paid to Christmas celebrations as they believed them to be *"encouraging gluttony, drunkenness, sexual licence and public disorder"*, banning it altogether in 1647 along with Easter and Whitsun.

Christmas as we know it was hugely influenced by people such as Charles Dickens and Prince Albert who reintroduced many customs from "Merrie England" such as mince pies, holly, ivy, mistletoe and hospitality to our neighbours. Prince Albert famously introduced the Christmas tree from his native Germany, and Father Christmas began to take centre stage. These "upper class" customs took a while to filter down to the poorer people in Victorian England and only really became the norm after World War II.

YULE GINGERBREAD FIZZING BATH BOMBS

Cinnamon and ginger are warming, as well as being antibacterial, antifungal and anti-inflammatory, and will leave your bathroom smelling amazing. Bicarbonate of soda is soothing for the skin, citric acid helps to remove dead skin cells and the fizz is just great fun!

INGREDIENTS

300 g food-grade bicarbonate of soda

100 g citric acid

2 tsp cinnamon powder

2 tsp ginger powder

Organic witch hazel in a spray bottle (available online)

Rubber gloves

METHOD

Wearing rubber gloves, combine all the dry ingredients together in a large bowl.

Spray small amounts of witch hazel into the bowl stirring constantly. Add more witch hazel until the mixture resembles wet sand and holds together when you squeeze it.

Press into a gingerbread man mould if you have one, or just form into balls with your hands.

Allow to dry, then store in a cool, dry place.

Drop into warm bath water to enjoy the scents of Yule!

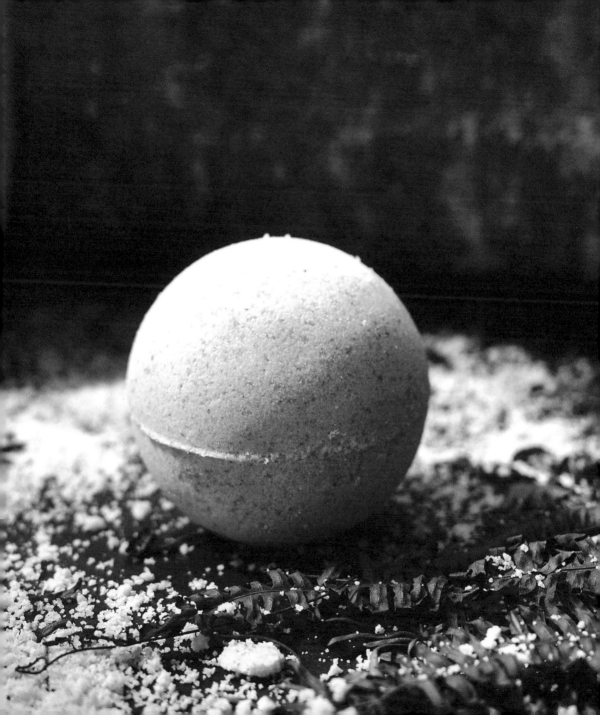

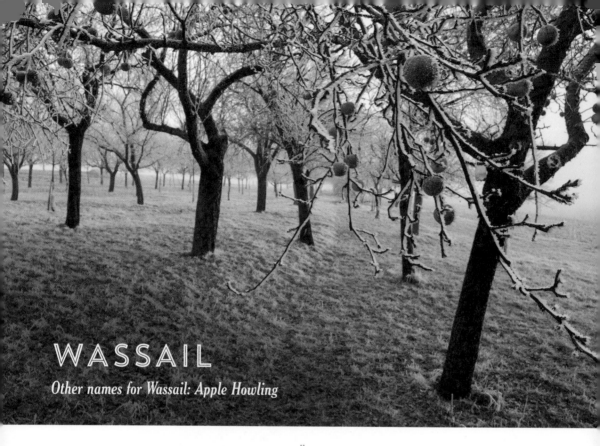

WASSAIL

Other names for Wassail: Apple Howling

HISTORY: Wassailing originated in Anglo-Saxon times and is carried out between Christmas Day and Twelfth Night. It prepares the trees for the coming year by awakening their spirit, ensuring they bear fruit. The spirit was believed to live in the oldest tree in the orchard and this particular tree is the centre of attention for the ceremony – in Somerset the spirit is known as "The Apple Tree Man". A wassail king and queen led the celebrations and were followed by the whole village, who were keen to join in with the noisy revelry. The wassailers process from orchard to orchard, making as much noise as possible: bashing pots and pans, firing shotguns, shouting and singing in order to scare away any wicked demons and awaken the sleeping tree spirit. All would gather around the oldest tree and watch the wassail queen place a piece of cider-soaked bread into its branches. The wassail drink was traditionally a warm cider or ale with honey and spices with even the addition of an egg or two. This was passed around in a large bowl giving the traditional "Wassail" greeting as it went from person to person.

This rhyme comes from the book *Bygone Haslemere: A Short History of the Ancient Borough and Its Immediate Neighbourhood from Earliest Times* by Ernest W. B. Swanton (1914):

"Here stands the good old
apple tree, stand fast root
Every little twig bear an apple big
Hats full, caps full, and three
score sacks full
Hip! Hip! Hurrah!"

Any leftover cider was thrown at the tree and, just to make sure that the spirit was awake, more gunshots would be fired into the branches. Wassailing wasn't just reserved for apple trees; plums and pears and any other fruit could be wassailed too.

It was believed that if the sun shone through the branches of the apple trees on Twelfth Night, there would be a bumper crop, but, just to be sure, 13 leaves from an apple tree were buried between its roots at the end of December. This number is believed to relate to Christ and his 12 disciples.

A second type of wassailing was known as "house visiting" and involved groups of young women dressed up with garlands and ribbons. They sang songs and recited rhymes spreading good wishes from door to door. In return, they hoped for food, drink or money. As with the wassailers in the orchard, the young ladies carried a bowl of spiced beer or cider described as "lamb's wool", as the addition of baked apples made it look white and fluffy.

House wassailing continued well into the Middle Ages, giving the feudal lord of the manor the opportunity to demonstrate how generous and charitable he was to the poor workers on his estate. Some wassailers carried a box containing two dolls, one to represent Baby Jesus, the other to represent the Virgin Mary. These were covered by a white cloth and could be shown, for a fee, to the householders while the others sang a festive song.

SPICED WASSAIL CIDER

Too delicious to save just for wassailing, this warm spicy alcoholic drink will warm you up on the coldest of winter days. For a non-alcoholic version, replace the cider with local cloudy apple juice.

INGREDIENTS

1 litre medium dry cider

200 g soft brown sugar

12 whole cloves

4 cinnamon sticks

1 apple, thinly sliced

METHOD

In a large saucepan, combine all the ingredients and bring to the boil while stirring to dissolve the sugar.

Simmer for 20–30 minutes and serve hot.

Wassail!

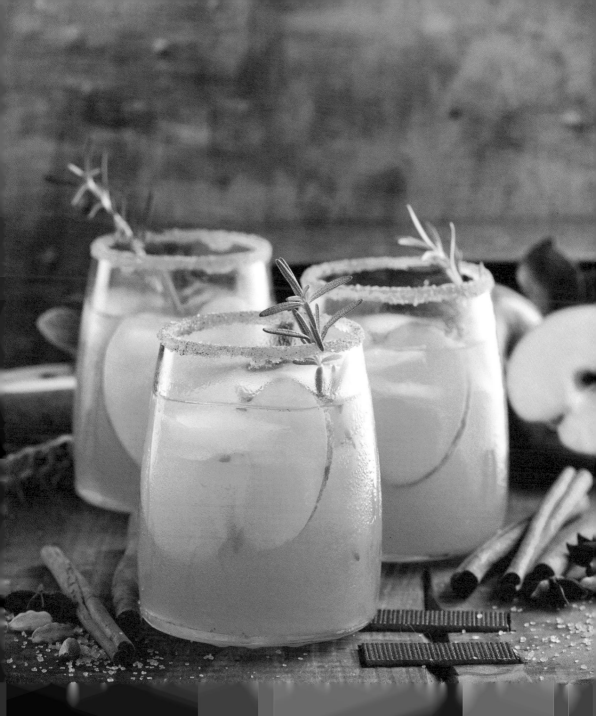

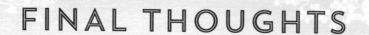

FINAL THOUGHTS

I hope this book has piqued your interest and will become a trusted companion when you go out into your local countryside to identify and forage for hedgerow treasures. Knowing the properties and uses for hedgerow plants opens up a wonderful new approach to healing common ailments. Once you begin your journey of discovery in the hedgerows looking for berries and flowers, you'll soon become obsessed with identifying more and more plants and researching the wonderful history and folklore attached to them. Several elderly villagers tell me that they "couldn't get through the winter coughs and colds" without their regular supply of elderberry rob (see page 74 for recipe), which I am only too happy to provide for them. As a family, we always look to nature first to safely treat minor ailments, of course consulting a medical practitioner for anything more serious.

Sadly, these days, our ancient hedgerows, which contribute hugely to the local biodiversity, are under constant threat from developers. This impacts dramatically on the local wildlife population who rely heavily on hedgerows, not just for food but for a safe corridor to journey through. Just by reading this book, I hope that it has made you more aware of the wonderful free resources that are available in the hedgerow. Maybe you'll be inspired to help to protect it and pass down the fascinating folklore to your children and your children's children.

Christine Iverson, *The Hedgerow Apothecary*

Image Credits

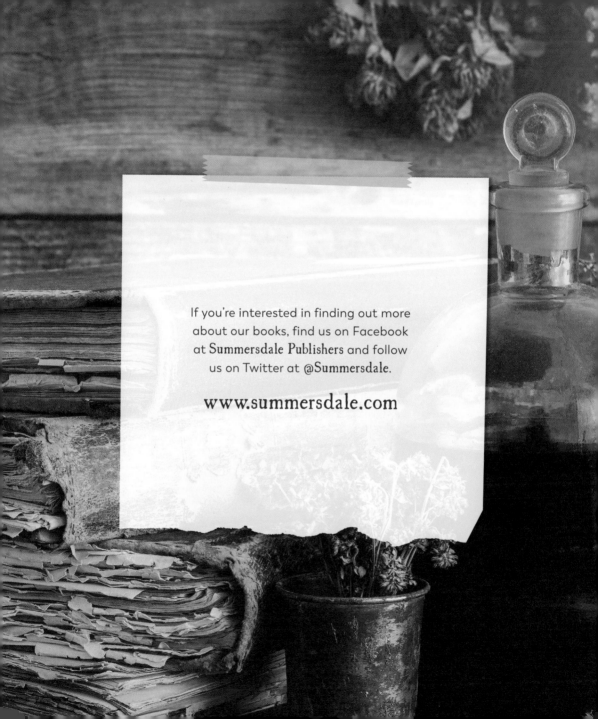

If you're interested in finding out more about our books, find us on Facebook at Summersdale Publishers and follow us on Twitter at @Summersdale.

www.summersdale.com

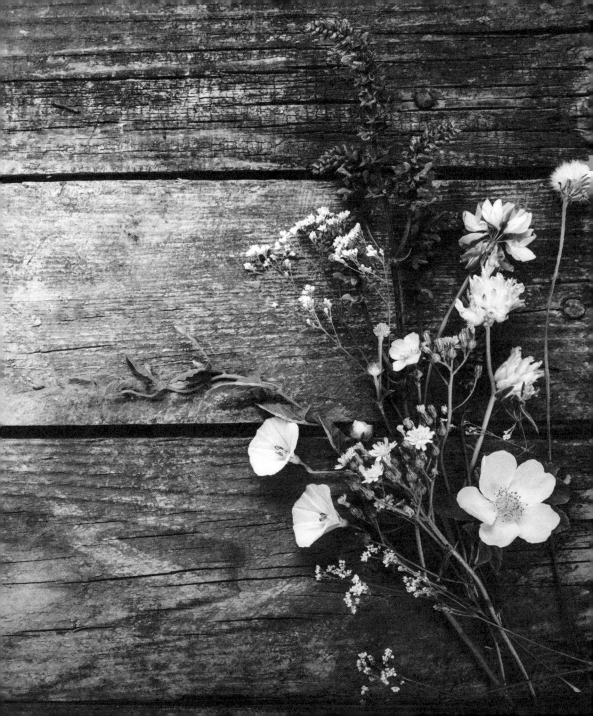

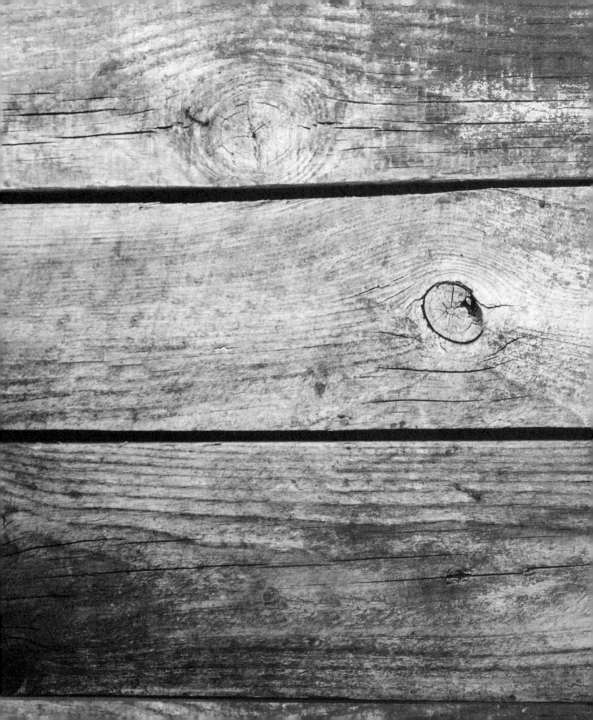